Healthcare Interpreting Explained

Healthcare Interpreting Explained is the first comprehensive, user-friendly book on the practice of medical/healthcare interpreting. Written by a leading world authority and drawing on research carried out in Europe, the United States, Australia and Asia, this process-focused text goes beyond terms and concepts to cover medical discourse, ethics and protocol, professionalization, cognitive factors, problem-solving strategies, assessment and more. Including summaries, tasks, further reading and a range of real-world examples, as well as audio files on the Translation Studies Portal, this is the essential text for all students and practicing interpreters in the areas of medical and healthcare interpreting.

Claudia V. Angelelli is Chair in Multilingualism and Communication at Heriot-Watt University (Edinburgh campus), UK, Emeritus Professor of Spanish Linguistics at San Diego State University, USA, and Visiting Professor at Beijing University of Foreign Studies, China. Her research lies at the intersection of sociolinguistics, applied linguistics and translation and interpreting studies. She is the sole author of *Medical Interpreting and Cross-cultural Communication* (2004) and *Revisiting the Interpreter's Role* (2004). She served as President and Vice President for the American Translation and Interpreting Studies Association and as Director for the American Translators Association. She was the World Project Leader for ISO 13611 Standards on Community Interpreting (PSI), approved as the first ISO Standard on community interpreting/PSI. She co-authored *The California Standards for Healthcare Interpreters: Ethical Principles, Protocols, and Guidance on Roles and Intervention* (2002). She has extensive experience as a freelancer and consultant in translation and community interpreting/PSI.

Translation Practices Explained
Series Editor: Kelly Washbourne

Translation Practices Explained is a series of coursebooks designed to help self-learners and students on translation and interpreting courses. Each volume focuses on a specific aspect of professional translation and interpreting practice, usually corresponding to courses available in translator- and interpreter-training institutions. The authors are practicing translators, interpreters, and/or translator or interpreter trainers. Although specialists, they explain their professional insights in a manner accessible to the wider learning public.

Each volume includes activities and exercises designed to help learners consolidate their knowledge, while updated reading lists and website addresses will also help individual learners gain further insight into the realities of professional practice.

Titles in the series:

Introduction to Court Interpreting 2e
Holly Mikkelson

Note-Taking for Consecutive Interpreting 2e
A Short Course
Andrew Gillies

Consecutive Interpreting
A Short Course
Andrew Gillies

Healthcare Interpreting Explained
Claudia V. Angelelli

For more information on any of these and other titles, or to order, please go to www.routledge.com/Translation-Practices-Explained/book-series/TPE

Additional resources for Translation and Interpreting Studies are available on the Routledge Translation Studies Portal: http://cw.routledge.com/textbooks/translationstudies

Healthcare Interpreting Explained

Claudia V. Angelelli

Routledge
Taylor & Francis Group
LONDON AND NEW YORK

First published 2019
by Routledge
2 Park Square, Milton Park, Abingdon, Oxon, OX14 4RN

and by Routledge
52 Vanderbilt Avenue, New York, NY 10017

Routledge is an imprint of the Taylor & Francis Group, an informa business

British Library Cataloguing-in-Publication Data
A catalogue record for this book is available from the British Library

Library of Congress Cataloging-in-Publication Data
Names: Angelelli, Claudia (Claudia V.), author. | Degueldre, Christian, co-author.
Title: Healthcare interpreting explained / Claudia V. Angelelli.
Description: First edition. | New York, NY : Routledge, [2019] | Series: Translation practices explained | Includes bibliographical references and index. |
Identifiers: LCCN 2019002896 (print) | LCCN 2019005889 (ebook) | ISBN 9781315310978 (E-book) | ISBN 9781138232945 (hardback) | ISBN 9781138232952 (pbk.)
Subjects: LCSH: Medicine—Translating. | Health facilities—Translating services.
Classification: LCC R119.5 (ebook) | LCC R119.5 .A528 2019 (print) | DDC 610.1/4—dc23
LC record available at https://lccn.loc.gov/2019002896

ISBN: 978-1-138-23294-5 (hbk)
ISBN: 978-1-138-23295-2 (pbk)
ISBN: 978-1-315-31097-8 (ebk)

Typeset in Times New Roman
by Apex CoVantage, LLC

Visit the eResources: www.routledge.com/9781138232952.

To my mother, *Nenucha*.

Your love, I will always feel; our laughs, I will always cherish.

Contents

Figures

Permissions

For specific permissions to reproduce five copyrighted texts, I thank:

- Gallaudet University Press, for the use of parts of Angelelli, C. (2014). "'Uh. . . I Am Not Understanding You at All': Constructing (Mis)Understanding in Provider/Patient-Interpreted Medical Encounters." In Metzger, M. *Investigations in Healthcare Interpreting.* Washington, DC: Gallaudet University Press, 2014.
- Springer.com (*Journal of General Internal Medicine*), for the story of Gricelda Zamora in Chen, A. H., Youdelman, M. K., Brooks, J. "The Legal Framework for Language Access in Healthcare Settings: Title VI and Beyond." *Journal of General Internal Medicine.* 2007;22 (Suppl 2):362–367. doi:10.1007/s11606-007-0366-2.
- Department of Health and Human Services (Victoria State Government 2018), for the article "Road and Traffic Safety for Children"
- Chen, A. H., Youdelman, M. K., Brooks, J. "The Legal Framework for Language Access in Healthcare Settings: Title VI and Beyond." *Journal of General Internal Medicine.* 2007;22 (Suppl 2):362–367. doi:10.1007/s11606-007-0366-2.
- Purdue OWL, for the definition of "Paraphrase" at https://owl.english.purdue.edu/owl/owlprint/619/

Every effort has been made to contact copyright holders. Please advise the publisher of any errors or omissions, and these will be corrected in subsequent editions.

About this book

Healthcare Interpreting Explained was inspired by the increasing needs of a linguistically diverse population accessing healthcare, as well as by the increasing number of issues faced by societies trying to accommodate the constantly fluctuating communicative needs of their diverse members. The focus of this book is on services related to healthcare and health education. New technologies, shrinking budgets, changes in budget allocations, geographic displacement, medical tourism, tensions between supply and demand of qualified interpreters, language access and language provision, right to language and linguistic discrimination all come together and play a part in healthcare interpreting. *Healthcare Interpreting Explained* is precisely about all of this.

This book is framed by the conceptualization of interpreting as both an act of communication and a situated practice. As in any act of communication, all parties to the interpreted communicative event contribute and play a part in both constructing meaning and/or reciprocal (mis)understanding of it. They have their own ways of communicating and they may or may not be proficient in the ways of communicating of others. In addition, all parties bring their own beliefs, traditions and *habitus* to the interpreted communicative event, in addition to their own social factors such as their age, education, ethnicity, gender, race and social class, which have a bearing on communication. As a situated practice, healthcare interpreting cannot be considered in isolation from the constraints imposed by the setting in which it occurs. It needs to be considered in its context. This also means that while there are many interpreting universals across the settings in which interpreting is practiced (e.g., conference, court or community interpreting, to name just a few), we focus on medical/healthcare interpreting as a situated practice, meaning we account for the uniqueness of the healthcare setting.

Healthcare Interpreting Explained is grounded in research. It is the product of many years of conducting studies in a variety of healthcare settings in various countries, including Argentina, Australia, Canada, China, Germany, Greece, Italy, Mexico, Spain, the United Kingdom and the United States. Throughout the book we use the results of empirical studies to illustrate the examples. However, because we are discussing stakeholders in abstract and representing many parts of the world, some degree of generalization is unavoidable. The bilingual healthcare encounters I observed and accessed either directly, or through interpreting, have provided the data to illustrate the issues we discuss in various chapters. This book is descriptive. All claims made in it are supported with evidence. It is not based on theoretical assumptions or prescriptions of what a practice should be like for the professionals/practitioners involved in it. This book focuses on healthcare interpreting as a field of specialization and inquiry in its own right. As such, it looks at a continuum of professionalism/practice. In this continuum we observe qualified professional medical interpreters on one end and non-professionals on the other; and a diverse and fluid middle ground populated with interpreters from other specializations crossing over to medical, recent graduates from interpreting programs, bilinguals with no experience but with a drive to help others, in addition to family members and friends who step up to the plate when no qualified interpreter is available. To protect confidentiality and privacy of participating informants in research studies that inform this book, all names of persons, locations and organizations are pseudonyms.

Healthcare interpreting, also called medical interpreting, does not enjoy the same status around the world. While in some countries medical interpreting is considered a profession and there are opportunities for education in interpreting as well as established professional associations that offer specific training in areas such as ethics or medical terminology, there are other countries in which medical interpreting is less developed. This does not mean that the need is not there or is not met by other means. My hope is that this book contributes to raise awareness about this professional practice as well as about the need to develop a cadre of professional medical interpreters who can provide users of non-societal languages with access to healthcare.

Using this book

Healthcare Interpreting Explained is designed to introduce readers to the knowledge and skills necessary to perform as medical interpreters. In my extensive journey of teaching at school, university and continuing education levels through classes, workshops or seminars in traditional classrooms, online and blended environments, I have embraced learner-centered approaches. This book is no exception. In my teaching and mentoring, I have guided my work by an adapted version of Maimonides' quote: "Give a learner a fish and you feed her for a day; teach a learner to fish and you feed her for a lifetime." *Healthcare Interpreting Explained* is rooted in this philosophy.

As it will become evident to the reader, when the parties who need to communicate do not share a language (in addition to having different views on well-being, health, illness, life and death), the interpreter bridges not only technical terms, cultures or emotions but also ways of speaking about them. Interpreting is not just about isolated words; it is about ways of speaking. The ways in which providers and patients communicate in a hospital or any other healthcare setting (e.g. a day clinic, an operating theater, the accidents and emergency department or a physiotherapy session) about issues is different. These different ways of speaking in addition to using different languages result in a complex communicative situation. Qualified medical interpreters resolve these situations and enable communication. They can do this as a result of their education (i.e. knowledge, skills and reflection), their professional judgment and their understanding of the context. This book offers readers tips and tools to build knowledge of medical topics and context. It also provides them the time and space for reflective learning.

Healthcare Interpreting Explained can be used in different ways. It can be used as a textbook in a classroom/online medical interpreting course; it can serve as an introduction to the field; and it can be used as a whole or as individual chapters/sections. For example, Chapter 1 can be used in an introductory class to give learners an opportunity to explore the profession of medical interpreting. Chapters 5 and 6 can be used in any interpreting class to introduce readers to basic skills in interpreting across settings. Readers will find a variety of activities that will help them develop interpreting skills such as anticipation, active listening, paraphrasing, split attention, multitasking and note-taking. They will also find data, discussions and readings to familiarize themselves with several aspects of the practice they are about to embrace. Readers will find that every claim made is supported by empirical evidence and, most importantly, they will distinguish supported claims and facts from opinions and experience and learn what is useful for them in each of these.

This book (whether used as a whole or as individual chapters or sections as described below) is aimed at a variety of readers who, for different reasons, may wish to explore the intricacies of healthcare interpreting:

- Advanced undergraduates and postgraduate students in translation, interpreting, mediation or cross-cultural communication;
- Practicing interpreters crossing over from other specializations in interpreting (e.g. court/legal, educational);
- Junior teachers and practitioners in the field of language teaching and language-service management, interpreting and mediation;
- Bilingual healthcare staff who may be asked to assist with interpreting tasks;
- Policy makers focusing on issues of access to healthcare on the part of users of non-societal language (i.e. linguistic minorities).

Healthcare Interpreting Explained contains eight chapters. Chapter 1 begins by introducing us to the field. It provides us with an overview of the professional practice, where it occurs, who provides it, how it is regulated, what it means to belong to an association and so forth. It also presents the different terms used to refer to medical interpreting and medical interpreters as well as opportunities for education. The professionalization of this practice is also discussed.

In Chapter 2 we learn about healthcare organizations, their context and their cultures. We examine the stakeholders in the organizations (providers, administrators) and the medical encounter (providers, patients, family members/friends), their responsibilities and roles. We learn about language access in various parts of the world and if language access is protected or mandated by law. Chapter 2 helps us gain an understanding of the physical setting in which medical interpreting generally occurs and how different cultures/languages interact.

Chapter 3 zooms in to interpreted medical communication and suggests a more comprehensive approach to medical interpreting. We shift our conceptualization of medical interpreting from terms to ways of speaking, from decontextualized assignments to a situated practice, and from the interpreter as an individual provider to a member of the healthcare team. Chapter 3 proposes to look at the medical encounter as a communicative event. This helps us describe and analyze the different parts of a medical interview as well as the different individuals who play a role in it.

In Chapter 4 we zoom even further in to look at the interaction, the communicative event. We pay special attention to the content and the form of communication. We look at the openings, closings and body of a conversation and how interpreters position themselves. We study what the provider and patient say and how they say it, and we look at how the interpreter handles the content and the form. We learn from experienced interpreters how they work with content and form, and how they solve misunderstandings when two cultural viewpoints are at odds with each other. Given that mental health care is one of the most challenging areas in which medical interpreters work, we explore the issues and intricacies of this specific healthcare area in more detail.

Chapters 5 and 6 differ from the other chapters in both content and form. They focus on skills and their practice. Relevant exercises are scattered throughout the chapter rather than under the B, C and D sections. Receptive skills (e.g. language and register for comprehension of input, topic preparation, reading about and around a topic, anticipation, information processing and text analysis) are discussed and practiced in Chapter 5. Productive skills (e.g. public speaking and delivery, memory, note-taking, self-monitoring, sight translation, ability to navigate cultural gaps, interpersonal skills, research skills and skills associated with technological competence) are in Chapter 6.

In Chapter 7 we explore the role of the medical interpreter, its evolution throughout time, and the discrepancy between the role as perceived by interpreters, by providers and by patients and the role as it emerges from research or as the result of prescriptive views. We problematize the blind transfer of interpreters' roles from other settings (e.g. conference or legal). We describe the continuum of roles played by interpreters working in the healthcare setting and the resulting communicative consequences.

Chapter 8 is about ethics and ethical dilemmas faced by medical interpreters while doing their jobs. We start with comparing and contrasting personal and professional ethics. We then examine the overlapping set of ethical principles that meet at the medical encounter. We discuss the medical ethics, ethical rules and principles that govern administrators and other providers such as nurses, psychologists or interpreters. We look at dilemmas and ways of solving them.

In each of the chapters, the reader will find approximately the same structure and sections, with the exception of Chapters 5 and 6 explained above.

Section A includes an evidence-based discussion on the main topic and subtopics of the chapter. It is followed by Section B, "Research, observe and reflect." In some chapters ROR is a guided activity to gain experience in observing systematically and learning from and reflecting on the observation; in others, ROR involves direct observations in public spaces, interviewing people and so forth. Section C, "Further Tasks," offers more space for practical activities on the topic or skill discussed in the chapter. Section D, "Journal Writing," gives the reader an opportunity to put all thoughts from the chapter into a reflexive piece. This may be in the form of a reflection on a question posed or a less guided type of reflection on a stated topic. The "References" section gives readers the complete references for sources used in the chapter. "Further Readings," provides readers with more readings on the topic, not discussed in the chapter but related to it. The reader may find in these readings videos, blogs and further useful information to complement the chapter discussion on the topic. At the end of the book, the reader will find a glossary of terms and an index.

My hope is that the topics researched and discussed in this book together with the practical activities followed by opportunities to reflect, analyze and further read/study will give the reader a thorough introduction to the exciting, demanding and rewarding field of healthcare interpreting. I also hope that when you complete the journey we are starting together, you will have become skilled in knowing where and how to look for the knowledge, the support and the practice or experience you need to succeed in your career. Bon voyage!

Acknowledgments

Many years of work and thoughts led to the writing of this book. I am, therefore, indebted to many people whose paths have crossed with mine at various stages of my journey through life as a practitioner, teacher and researcher. I wish to thank Mona Baker, who initially approached me with the idea for this book back in 2012 right before St. Jerome was acquired by Routledge. This book evolves from thoughts and perspectives which I first presented in the California Health Partnership and the Connecting World Collaborative Testing Project in 2003. I wish to thank colleagues and friends from the California Healthcare Interpreting Association, the National Council for Interpreters in Healthcare, Healthy House in Merced, the *Hablamos Juntos* network in the United States and the Healthcare Interpreting Network and Multilingual Corporation in Canada for the heated discussions as we were bridging theory, research and practice in what was considered at the time an incipient field.

I first discovered the uniqueness of the medical setting as a child of two healthcare providers in Argentina. At an early age, I visited the hospitals in which my mother or father worked during public holidays and weekends, when my parents were on duty. Later I returned to the same hospitals as a university graduate to teach English and translate for their colleagues who to date are like members of our extended family. Having family members as insiders allowed me to discover the challenges of hospitals and healthcare organizations as places of work. I returned several times for the last 30 years to visit and observe provider-patient communication in various specialties. All of these experiences have paved the way for me to navigate hospitals comfortably and join communities of discourse of healthcare providers with some understanding of the challenges they face. For all the lessons learned, and for holding my hand as I learned, I will always be grateful to both my parents and my extended, "adopted" family.

This book would not have been possible without the participants (patients, families, interpreters, providers and administrators) of the studies I have conducted across languages on medical/healthcare interpreting, cross-cultural communication and access to healthcare in Argentina, Australia, Belgium, China, Germany, Greece, Italy, Spain, the United Kingdom and the United States. To these participants goes my highest debt of gratitude. The findings of my own empirical studies from the last 20 years – as well as those from colleagues working in this field – have paved the way for empirically based learning, teaching and testing of medical/healthcare interpreting.

Equally important has been the support received from various foundations and universities who partially funded my work in this area. Specifically, I wish to express my gratitude to:

- The California Endowment, under the directorship of Ignatius Bao, for the funding received to explore language proficiency, register and medical-interpreter readiness in Cantonese, English, Hmong and Spanish (2001–2003).
- The California Healthcare Interpreting Association for the funding received to study California healthcare interpreter's perceptions and beliefs on the CHIA Code of Ethics and Standards of Practice.
- The Robert Wood Johnson Foundation for the funding received through *Hablamos Juntos* (We Speak Together) under the directorship of Yolanda Partida, to adapt my work on language proficiency, register and medical interpreting skills from California and implement it at a national level in the United States (2002–2004).
- The European Union Directorate General Translation (Josep Bonet-Heras, Head of Professional and Organizational Development Unit and Catherine Vieilledent-Monfort, Coordinator of Studies on Translation and Multilingualism at the DGT) for funding received in 2014–2015 to study translation and interpreting provision in cross-border healthcare in the European Union in the framework of Directive 2011/24/EU.
- Hamburg University and the seminars I attended as a Visiting Scientist for MedIntin, led by Prof. Bernd Meyer and Kristin Bullrich in 2010.
- Macquarie University, where I spent my sabbatical in 2010 and returned to lead a project with Dr. Helen Slatyer to study the role of medical interpreters in rural and urban healthcare settings in Australia 2012.
- The Robert Wood Johnson Foundation for the funding received through *Hablamos Juntos* (We Speak Together) under the directorship of Yolanda Partida to adapt my work on language proficiency, register and medical interpreting skills and implement it at a national level in the United States in 2002–2004.

Access to observations, interviews and data collection from medical encounters, meetings and documents from healthcare organizations in rural and urban areas as well as information and participation in professional organizations inform every section of this book. Procedures to protect participants in studies that inform this book were obtained and appropriate protocols for ethics approval were filed. However, access is not guaranteed by following rules. It requires human effort, support and trust. Access may not have been possible without the support I received from many organizations, institutions, associations, patients and healthcare and interpreting professionals who will remain anonymous and to whom I will always be indebted. I also want to specifically thank the following colleagues and project collaborators who were instrumental in opening doors for me. Without their help and contacts, it would have been difficult for me to approach healthcare organizations, policy makers, practitioners, leaders of professional associations and teachers in parts of the world in which I was working on a temporary basis. From countries (in alphabetical order) I wish to thank: Argentina: Dr. Hugo Alume, Dr. Angela Rizzo de Angelelli, Dr. Lucho Koss, Dra Rosa Nuñez and Dra Valeria Pachioli; Australia: Dr. Helen Slatyer; Belgium: Christian Degueldre and Dr. Charlie Cuypers; China: Dr. Cheng Zhan; Germany: Feyza Ervin and Prof. Bernd Meyer; Greece: Dr. Ana Chitta, Dr. Pannagiota Karanasiou, Dr. Evengelia Kouremenou and Dimitra Strafilia; Italy: Prof. Claudio Baraldi and Prof. Laura Gavioli; Spain: Dr. María Jesus Blasco Mayor and Dr. Maribel de Pozo Triviño.

Special thanks go to my own students and those from various universities in the world with whom I have engaged in challenging discussions during regular courses, workshops or lectures. Their questions and comments as well as their feedback from specific activities I have piloted with them have been extremely insightful. Many colleagues from the universities and associations where I have worked have enhanced my thoughts on medical interpreting throughout these years. I would like to specially thank Tanya Croman, Ryan DeJonge, Doris Fernandez del Pozo, Lauren Machta, Antonella Nardella, Anaid Stere Lugo and Despina Sourli. Discussions in meetings and conference presentations have allowed me to exchange views with researchers, practitioners, students and teachers coming to healthcare interpreting from applied linguistics, communication, interpreting studies and linguistic anthropology. To all of them (too many to mention by name) for their comments and questions, I will always be grateful.

Friends and family have been extremely supportive throughout the writing of this book. They have patiently tolerated my stories and questions as well as my absences from important events. I wish to thank all of them for their patience and love. In particular, I wish to thank my good friend and professional singer, Doc (Scott Whitaker), for making a recording of an adapted health broadcast. His laughs, friendship and professionalism are gifts I treasure.

A big debt of gratitude goes to Christian Degueldre, my husband and experienced interpreter educator, professional interpreter/translator and co-author of two chapters. Writing a manuscript of this type occurs during an extended period of time during which life happens. During the writing of this manuscript, I had a serious family emergency which lasted over two years. Life went off-balance and my writing time was severely challenged. Christian understood the increasing pressure I was under as well as the tensions arising from being an only child and managing healthcare across countries. He encouraged me to persevere in almost impossible conditions because it was important for me to see this book in print.

And last but not least, I am indebted for the professionalism and compassion with which the Routledge editorial team handled my emergency and encouraged me to pursue a late submission. Without the support and kindness of Louisa Semlyen, Senior Publisher, Routledge English and Linguistics; Kelly Washbourne, Series Editor and Hannah Rowe and Eleni Steck, Editorial Assistants this project may not have come to fruition.

1 Introduction to the professional practice of healthcare interpreting

GOALS

In this chapter we will:

- Familiarize ourselves with the concept of healthcare interpreting.
- Review some of the educational opportunities available for healthcare interpreters (from formal education to professional development) and their certification/accreditation.
- Problematize the notions of professional practice and professionalism in various parts of the world.

LEARNING OUTCOMES

By successfully completing this chapter, we will be able to:

- Compare and contrast healthcare interpreting in various areas of the world (in terms of historical background, educational opportunities, challenges and certification).
- Understand the concept of professionalism, requirements of professions and the difference between training and professional developments.
- Contextualize healthcare interpreting in legislation related to equality, access to information and patients' rights.

This chapter presents an overview of the professional practice of healthcare interpreting. It discusses the work performed by professional and non-professional healthcare interpreters. By acknowledging the realities of the field, we explore a continuum of aptitude, knowledge and professionalism. In addition, we study the practice and the existing tension between supply and demand. We review other terms that are used to refer to professional and non-professional interpreters working in healthcare. We examine definitions that are used to refer to the healthcare interpreter. We then focus on the educational opportunities available to healthcare interpreters as well as training possibilities. We problematize the term training and education. We look at the certification/accreditation opportunities and the professionalism of healthcare interpreters as well as their opportunities for professional development/continuing education.

A. Introduction to healthcare interpreting

Healthcare interpreting occurs when a provider and a patient need to communicate and do not share a language. In our ever-changing and diverse societies, multilingualism has become the norm rather than the exception. Some areas of the world are undoubtedly more diverse than others. However, we could safely state that monolingual or monocultural societies are becoming extinct. In many places of the world, there are groups of people who do not access the language of the society in which they are immersed. These groups are called linguistic minorities. The language of the society is called the societal language. Some countries have one societal language (e.g. France) and others have more (e.g. Belgium, which has Flemish, French and German). Linguistic minorities can only access healthcare services through healthcare interpreters because they cannot access the societal language. There are different situations that lead people to become a linguistic minority in a country. Based on life circumstances, individuals become a linguistic minority as a group or as an individual. Here are some examples of how people become part of a linguistic minority:

- A person may be in a relationship with another person from a different country/region and move to be reunited. Two people have a language in common; they can communicate with each other but they cannot access the societal language of either.
- People may migrate and settle in a country and they cannot access the language of their host country.
- People may be born in a country but cannot access the societal language of that country (e.g. deaf and hard of hearing individuals can access sign language but not spoken language).
- People may migrate to pursue better economic opportunities or start a different career.
- People may suffer from adverse political, social or economic conditions in their own country and decide to leave it behind.
- People may be touring a country without being able to speak the language. While traveling, they may need to access healthcare and they are not able to communicate.
- People may go abroad with the specific goal of seeking medical treatment and they cannot access the target country language.
- People can belong to original/indigenous groups in a country and never have learned the societal language.
- People may take refuge or seek asylum in a country in which they cannot access the societal language.

- People can become displaced as a consequence of a natural disaster, war, political upheaval, guerrillas, persecution (political, religious or gender-based), sexual and commercial exploitation, or as victims of human trafficking.

In addition to traditional reasons for which people move or become displaced, current regional agreements among culturally and linguistically diverse areas (e.g. the European Union or the Association of South East Asian Nations) result in more frequent communication on healthcare across borders and in higher numbers of mobile patients. This means increased opportunities for patients (provided they can afford to be mobile, both physically as well as financially) to pursue healthcare in a different country/member state and avoid long waiting times for specific treatment or surgeries in their own countries. Mobility triggers the need for communication across languages and cultures, as diverse patients may seek care in a country/region whose societal language they do not understand. This is why the need for professional healthcare interpreting is more pressing than ever.

In healthcare encounters in which a language is not shared by provider and patient(s), interpreters step in to meet the communicative needs of diverse people who interact via spoken or signed communication. A healthcare interpreter is the person who delivers language-related services to clients/patients who cannot access the societal language. The healthcare interpreter enables the patient to communicate with doctors, nurses and other **medical** staff. Healthcare interpreters may be employed by healthcare/medical organizations (e.g. National Health Service), private or public hospitals or **interpreting agencies**, or they may freelance or choose to operate their own businesses.

In some European countries (e.g. United Kingdom, Spain), healthcare interpreters are called public-service interpreters. A healthcare/public-service interpreter is essential for linguistic minorities to exercise their right to communicate and access services.[1] It is through healthcare interpreting that health and social institutions fulfill their obligations of providing health-related services to entitled linguistic minorities. "Regardless of geographic location (e.g. urban or rural areas) or language (spoken or sign), speakers of the societal language and linguistic minorities communicate effectively, deliver and access healthcare services through healthcare interpreters" (ISO 13611 2014).

Healthcare interpreting and healthcare interpreters by any other name . . .

Healthcare interpreting (HI) is also referred to as **medical interpreting**. It is also called **public-service interpreting** (PSI, as discussed above) in many European Union member states. Sometimes **liaison interpreting** or **dialogue interpreting** are terms used to refer to HI. It falls under the umbrella of community interpreting because it refers to interpreting that occurs within the community (rather than in an organization, a company, at a conference or in a court of law) and has a community member as one of the participants. Generally, this community member is part of a linguistic minority (e.g. a Polish speaker in Scotland, a Hmong speaker in the United States or a Auslan signer in Australia). As a consequence, this community member has limited or no access to the societal language of the place in which the member is trying to access services (e.g. education, health, government programs). Because in the European Union the term "community interpreting" was used for interpreters working in the European Community (e.g. at the European Parliament or Commission in Brussels), the term PSI has been preferred in Europe more than anywhere else.

Healthcare interpreting can be defined as a

> special type of interpreting that facilitates communication between users and providers of health services who do not share the same language (either spoken or signed). It occurs mainly in settings such as hospitals, clinics, and doctor offices and involves the communication of signed, verbal and non-verbal messages in real time. The language of one user group (the provider) is mainly the/a societal language of the country. The language of the patient is the non-societal language, i.e., the language of a specific ethnic/linguistic group. Healthcare interpreting serves the latter user group to ensure their access to healthcare services.
>
> (Angelelli 2014: 574)

Other related terms

In addition to healthcare interpreting, the following terms are used to refer to related concepts to intercultural/linguistic communication in healthcare, including mental health. To ensure we have a shared understanding, during our journey learning about healthcare interpreting we begin by looking at some concepts, trace their origin and ensure we can differentiate among these terms.

Language/linguistic and cultural mediation: In multilingual and multicultural societies, this term refers to a possible solution for migrants' inclusion in institutional services (Baraldi 2017). In the language industry, the term "cultural (and linguistic) mediator" refers to a person who assists a person or a group to communicate more effectively across languages and cultures. This is deemed necessary because one may not understand the societal language at all, or may have difficulty comprehending certain terms or concepts as they may not exist in one's own language/culture, or one may be dealing with situations or ideas with which one is not familiar. The *Common European Framework of Reference for Languages* (2001) refers to this specific type of mediation as inclusive of interpreting and translation among other tasks a cultural mediator may perform. It states:

> the written and/or oral activities of mediation make communication possible between persons who are unable, for whatever reason, to communicate with each other directly. Translation or interpretation, a paraphrase, summary or record, provides for a third party a (re)formulation of a [spoken or written] source text to which this third party does not have direct access. Mediating

> language activities – (re)processing an existing text – occupy an important place in the normal linguistic functioning of our societies.
>
> (2001: 14)

The language/linguistic mediator may or may not have credentials in healthcare interpreting or hold a degree in a related field of languages or intercultural communication.

Bilingual: A person who can use two languages (e.g. Chinese/English bilingual). These languages may be at different or equal levels of proficiency. There is a misconception that bilingual individuals, on the basis of their bilingualism and without a relevant education in healthcare interpreting, can provide adequate language services. For bilinguals, the proficiency in each of their language varies along a continuum (Angelelli 2010a, 2010b). Differences are not only between the two languages (e.g. proficiency in both English and Chinese may not be similar; Chinese may be stronger or weaker than English), but also proficiency differs across skills (e.g. writing, listening, socio-cultural awareness) within each of the languages. The Chinese/English bilingual in our example may read and write better in English than in Chinese and may be strong in listening and speaking in Chinese. In other words, being bilingual does not mean being a balanced bilingual (Angelelli 2010a, 2010b), which appears to be the type of bilingualism discussed when referring to interpreting. Unfortunately, the parties most affected by the interpreting service lack the skills to judge its quality. They assume the person providing interpreting is doing an adequate job. As a consequence, the parties present may have a sense of security that effective communication is taking place when in reality they are not in a position to ascertain it.

Translator: A person transferring a written/video/electronic message from one language to another. There are differences between a translator and an interpreter. In addition to dealing with written language rather than spoken or sign, a translator has a certain amount of time allocated for the task, whereas an interpreter works in real time. In addition to the difference between written and oral/sign language, or to the task occurring in real life versus planned time, translation conceptualizes communication as information transfer, whereas interpreting conceptualizes communication as human interaction. This difference is essential, as will become evident through our discussion in various chapters of this book.

In addition to the terms above, qualifiers such as ad hoc, volunteer, untrained or non-certified are used to refer to persons acting as HIs to suggest that these individuals have had no formal education in HI and/or have not obtained certification. The qualifier *volunteer* implies that the person is not receiving payment in return for the services rendered (Evrin and Meyer 2016). The use of *ad hoc* suggests a person who may or may not be qualified and may or may not engage in healthcare interpreting frequently. In healthcare settings, these ad hoc interpreters are called dual-role translators/interpreters. The qualifier *dual-role*, in the healthcare context, refers to staff members in a healthcare organization (e.g. a lab technician or a nurse) who are bilingual and who are asked to perform tasks related to interpreting (or translation) for patients with whom they share a language. These requests to perform as interpreters are in addition to performing the work for which they are hired. Another qualifier used in healthcare to refer to these persons is *lay* (Hlavac 2011), as in lay interpreter.

Educational opportunities and certification/accreditation

Healthcare interpreting has evolved in terms of research and visibility, growing both as a field of study in its own right and as a recognized service, required in light of our linguistic diversity. Healthcare interpreting, however, is lagging behind in two important areas: education and professional recognition (which generally is evidenced by lower remuneration). In the next two sections we will discuss education of healthcare interpreters and then review professional recognition.

Education or training? Available options

Before exploring options, we should discuss the differences between the terms education and training, as they are not synonyms. Education involves acquiring knowledge about facts, events, values, beliefs, behaviors, general concepts, principles and so forth. Therefore, an education on healthcare interpreting may include learning about the profession, its practice, the context where it takes place, its history, its recognition, how it intersects with healthcare, how it is viewed in a healthcare organization, the main events in its development (e.g. publication of code of ethics, certification/accreditation exams), the ethics of the profession and common ethical dilemmas, what beliefs are held among clients about the role of the healthcare interpreter, who defines the role, what behaviors are favored, accepted and unaccepted, what triggers interpreter's behaviors, what the standards of practice are and so on. An education in healthcare interpreting also involves developing the research-based skills and knowledge-based practices expected to perform at various levels and contexts (to interpret in the emergency room, to interpret for psychotic patients, to interpret for a child with or without parents present, to sight-translate a consent form, to interpret using short consecutive, to interpret over the phone to one party at a time, to interpret over a speakerphone to two parties who are face-to-face and the interpreter present only through voice, to interpret on a video remote conference, etc.).

When pursuing educational opportunities in healthcare interpreting, one learns to understand, analyze, evaluate or contextualize concepts and knowledge. One also learns to distinguish between general and specific issues. For example, one learns to look at the big picture in which an issue is contextualized (e.g. the working conditions of the healthcare providers, their backgrounds and their interactions with patients, the working environment and the pressures/constraints it imposes on them). One also learns to consider the specifics of the issue at hand (how providers address a patient who needs to communicate with the help of an interpreter, how providers address the interpreter, how they accommodate the interpreting in their practice, etc.). The learning that takes place through the process of education enables a person to face future challenges and solve problems. It affords the person the time to reflect on new knowledge as it sinks in and interacts with previously acquired knowledge. This knowledge, together with skills and abilities, develops over time as one engages in reflexive learning and guided practice.

Training, on the other hand, refers to learning specific job-related skills, such as the protocol of a healthcare process (e.g. triage), the protocol used by interpreters to introduce the self as they start working, how to report the malfunctioning of a piece of remote equipment or an inappropriate behavior observed by the interpreter and so forth. Training is a common concept in human resources. It is task-oriented and skill-focused, thus it does not provide the depth and breadth needed for creative problem-solving, which is part of what bilingual healthcare communication requires. Without the benefits of an HI education, when a learner gets training it is important to contextualize the information obtained in training in the appropriate way. For example, attending training on medical terminology may provide learner access to terms that are important and necessary. Learners, however, need to be aware that terms are only one component of the medical discourse, of the ways in which healthcare professionals speak, with which healthcare interpreters have to familiarize themselves. Brief courses or seminars are offered on the ethics of the profession. As with healthcare terminology, ethics are important, but learners need to also be critical readers, to learn and question the origin and foundations of codes of ethics. This may not be achievable, for example, in a brief training session about the content and organization of a code.

Education available for interpreters

In HI, the need for education is real but it is also complex, and more often than not it is replaced by training. When one decides to pursue a career in HI and looks for educational opportunities, among other things, one considers the cost of education, the job market and the potential income. Across the world, formal opportunities for education in interpreting in general, and HI in particular, are not many. And those that exist have a different focus, as healthcare interpreting is not the most well-remunerated kind of interpreting, although it is definitely one of the most needed and rewarding. In the next sections we briefly discuss interpreting education opportunities available in different settings.

EDUCATION FOR HEALTHCARE INTERPRETERS

Currently, for HI there are no university programs specializing only in healthcare. HI seems to be subsumed under the umbrella of community interpreting or public-service interpreting. There is one master's program in Alcalá de Henares, Spain (Master's in Intercultural Communication, Public Service Interpreting and Translation), which offers more than one course in PSI. Another one-year Master's in Business and Public Service Interpreting and Translation Studies is offered at the University of Leeds, UK. Several courses on public service interpreting are taught in universities where translation, interpreting or linguistic/cultural mediation are taught. Some examples are the Middlebury Institute of International Studies at Monterey (California, USA), Heriot-Watt University and University of Surrey (Scotland and England, UK). Healthcare interpreters supplement their education with options such as continuing education seminars, professional development courses, preconference workshops and so forth, as discussed earlier. These may be online, blended or face-to face. However, such educational opportunities vary in quality (Kennen 2005).

Most of the courses offered by institutions (universities, community colleges) or organizations (hospitals, community agencies) devoted to the teaching of interpreters do not focus as much on the education of the individuals who facilitate communication across cultures as they do on the training of how to interpret. Regardless of the length (from 40 hour to an entire semester or year) or mode of instruction (face-to-face, distance learning or blended), courses are limited, narrow in scope and, for the most part, of a pragmatic nature. The focus is not on educating well-rounded interpreters as much as it is on training in specific areas, such as information-processing skills or terminology. While it would be pointless to argue that terminology is not relevant, it is not sufficient and should definitely not drive the curriculum of healthcare interpreting. A focus on decontextualized terminology, a bilingual list of terms stripped from the discourse in which they are embedded, may mislead students. Terminology and glossaries derive from ways of speaking in a contextualized setting. They are pieces of a whole. They need to be included as part of a curriculum but should not constitute the centerpiece. Once again, education gets confused with training. Reducing the education of healthcare interpreters (or any type of interpreter for that matter) to training (1) assumes that their knowledge of the field is sufficient enough for them to contextualize the newly acquired information and (2) provides a limited opportunity to focus specifically on an objective (e.g. tips on how to use portable equipment).

While all of these pieces are important, they are only specific pieces of a puzzle, the solution to which may not be as simple as just having access to a master's program in healthcare interpreting. Of course, such a program is not only desirable but would also guarantee recognition and professionalism of the field, which would definitely materialize into higher fees. But it cannot be a one-size-fits-all type of solution. Since healthcare interpreters could be "crossovers" from other settings, other paths of life (individuals with academic careers in other areas, such as conference interpreting, nursing or social work), education for healthcare interpreters needs to be flexible enough to accommodate competent bilingual individuals who may already possess a background in healthcare, interpreting or other areas of applied linguistics or intercultural communication. In this way, healthcare interpreting could become a specialization for those learners who wish to cross over into this profession. Meaningful testing in language proficiency (Angelelli 2007) would verify their language abilities are up to the demands of interpreting, and by learning about the specifics of healthcare interpreting, these individuals could gain knowledge in the areas necessary to complement the education they already possess.

EDUCATION FOR COURT OR COMMUNITY INTERPRETERS

There are more opportunities to study court interpreting than healthcare interpreting. Examples of countries in which university educational programs in court/legal interpreting can be found are Australia, Belgium, Canada, Mexico, United Kingdom and United States. In some countries, legal interpreting is a strand of legal translation and comparative law (e.g. Argentina, Spain). In addition to universities, several professional associations offer ongoing professional development courses about changes in legislation or on issues specific to the specialization (financial law, estate planning, etc.).

EDUCATION FOR CONFERENCE INTERPRETERS

In many countries, educational opportunities for interpreters are mostly focused on conference interpreting. Examples are Cameroon, Ghana and Mozambique in Africa; Argentina, Canada, Chile, Colombia, Mexico, United States or Uruguay, to name a few in the Americas; Belgium, France, Germany, Greece, Hungary, Italy, Latvia, Poland, Romania, Spain, Sweden and the United Kingdom, to name some European Union member states; China, Japan, South Korea, Taiwan and Thailand in Asia; Australia and New Zealand in Oceania; and Israel and Lebanon in the Middle East. In fact, there are 49 university members of CIUTI[2] on four continents. In addition, the International Association of Conference Interpreters (AIIC 2018) lists 87 schools in 15 regions covering 36 languages, in which conference interpreting is taught in several language combinations. The prevalence of conference interpreting in educational offerings is due to the need for communication in conference settings as well as the interpreter's potential income generation, compared to other forms of interpreting.

Conference interpreters work for political organizations (e.g. the European Union, the United Nations), for heads of state, business executives and other leaders, professionals, celebrities and so forth. In the meetings in which they work, the cost of interpreting is factored in, as the conference may not have the same results without professional interpreters. There appears to be a genuine concern for quality and professionalism on the part of conference interpreters. In spite of this, some AIIC members have reported that working conditions are not as generous as they were in the past (Angelelli 2004), especially when it comes to traveling conditions, resting time, per diem and so forth. In addition to the power of many of the speakers/organizations for whom conference interpreters work, there is the attention gained by the activity of conference interpreters. They work, most of the time, for an audience. Along a continuum of better to not so good remunerated interpreting jobs, we find conference interpreting leading the list, followed by court interpreting, followed by HI/PSI. As a consequence, it is not surprising to see educational opportunities for settings other than conferences to be fewer.

To sum up, in terms of education, if we paint a picture of healthcare interpreting offerings, whether within or outside a university, it does not look very different from what conference interpreting looked like in its inception. Immigration waves, economic forces or new legislation result in an imminent need for displaced linguistic minorities with limited proficiency in the societal language to access healthcare. By definition, linguistic minorities do not share equal or similar socio-economic status with users of the societal language. Differences between speakers who belong to different speech communities (Angelelli 2000) result in interactions where power differentials are extremely salient, such as those we observe in bilingual hospital encounters (and/or asylum-seeking interviews, court cases or teacher-parent conferences). Research questions about this practice, its practitioners and their education, which are essential to guiding pedagogy and understanding the underlying complexities of the interpreted communicative event in a medical setting (Angelelli 2000; Davidson 2001; Metzger 1999), are deferred to the market needs. Access to healthcare, however, cannot and should not wait, in the same way as right after World War II communication between heads of state could not wait. Therefore, today, as in the 1950s, education is reduced to training to cope with immediate needs.

Brief historical background of interpreter education

To understand the limited availability of educational opportunities for interpreting in general and for healthcare interpreting in particular, and the prevalence of training (based only on practice) versus well-rounded education, we trace the historical background of interpreter education. In so doing, we ask ourselves when, why or how did interpreting become part of higher education. In the early days (immediately after World War II), the need to educate interpreters was triggered by the need to ensure communication between heads of state or delegates of international organizations. Since the need was urgent, no time could be afforded to design a curriculum, to conduct research on best practices of education or to become familiar with competing theories that can guide and inform practice. Consequently, many of the curricular decisions were made based on the personal experience of those who practiced interpreting and then needed to pass along their practice to others.

Interestingly, however, if we consider the rise of patient mobility within a geographical area (e.g. Europe), as well as the increase of medical tourism in many countries, the senior/retiree communities of expatriates in various countries and the steady increase of displaced linguistic minorities in need to access healthcare, one may be shocked by the scarcity of educational offerings in HI. This means that educational offerings are not only related to the needs of the community but also to the level of income to be expected from each of these specializations – and in the case of healthcare interpreting, remuneration is still lagging behind. This is due to various reasons: (1) linguistic minorities are not as noticeable as heads of state or celebrities; (2) communication about health is a private matter and does not make news; it only matters to the participants; (3) as a consequence of limited educational opportunities, interpreters have limited access to advanced degrees which, generally, guarantee higher pay. Given all of this, the problem of professional recognition remains unsolved.

What is a professional healthcare interpreter?

Research-based pedagogy on healthcare interpreting has explored the minimum knowledge which an individual characterized as a professional in HI needs to have. This knowledge comes from at least six different areas: (1) information processing; (2) linguistic; (3) interpersonal; (4) professional ethics; (5) setting-specific; and (6) socio-cultural (Angelelli 2007). These six areas can either be found in one program or course or be offered as pieces of various programs or courses. Information-processing and linguistic areas are generally present in discussions about teaching interpreting, that is, how to transfer information from one language to another (we learn about these skills in Chapters 5 and 6). In addition to terminology, we need to become familiar with the ways of speaking in healthcare settings (area 5) which, as discussed above, means going beyond the use of specific terminology (we learn ways of speaking in Chapters 3 and 4). It may mean gaining background information, such as reading about or studying anatomy and physiology (Crezee 2013), understanding a medical interview (Drew and Heritage 1992) or mastering the most frequent expressions and terms that occur during a specific speech event (e.g. a provider-patient presurgical consultation). We learn about preparation for assignments, content and form of messages in Chapter 4.

In addition, we reflect about our roles and positioning during our work. We must be mindful of the agency we have as interpreters, how we interact (area 3) with others as we work and set or do not set boundaries between personal and professional. We must be aware of the responsibilities and duties that arise from our participation in interactions (area 4). Additionally, we go about our work, realizing its socio-cultural context (area 6), understanding interpreting is a situated practice and therefore we notice the impact that both the institution and society have on the interactions we broker.

It is evident that one should give serious consideration to healthcare interpreting education. While the path may not be linear, the opportunities exist. Gaining a well-rounded education in HI means understanding the issues at the macro and micro levels, as this book will show. At the macro level we need to become familiar with the profession and its practice as well as the underlying theory in which our practice is grounded, the work context (the setting), the stakeholders (the participants), the rules about language provision and access to healthcare by users of non-societal languages, the ethics of the profession in general and the workplace(s) (e.g. a hospital, a telephone interpreting company) in which we interpret in particular, and the ways of speaking in healthcare settings. At the micro level we need to become familiar with issues of the content and form of healthcare discourse in general and of interpreted healthcare discourse in particular. We also need to learn the skills to perform in a professional way. In the following chapters, we discuss each of these areas more at length.

Professional practice, profession and professionalism

Up until the 1990s, healthcare interpreting was perceived as a less prestigious variety of interpreting, practiced mostly by ad hoc interpreters. As an offshoot of community interpreting, healthcare interpreting went through the expected stages new disciplines go through (Mikkelson 1996). It was frowned upon by interpreters working in other settings who had pursued an education and worked hard to obtain recognition in their work. Since then, healthcare interpreting has been gaining recognition across other fields of inquiry. Evidence of this is the increasing number of:

1 Interdisciplinary funded projects, such as the program We Speak Together/ *Hablamos Juntos* of the Robert Wood Johnson Foundation (Moreno 2010), in which healthcare interpreting is a key player;
2 Academic publications in scholarly journals in other disciplines, such as Hilfinger Messias et al. (2009) in *Advances in Nursing Science*, Price (1975) in *Australian and New Zealand Journal of Psychiatry* and Woloshin et al. (1995) in *JAMA Network*;
3 Encyclopedia entries, such as Angelelli (2012) in the *Encyclopedia of Applied Linguistics*;
4 Statutes: In the United Kingdom, British Sign Language (Scotland) Act 2015 asp 11, which received Royal Assent on 22 October 2015. In Italy, the Turco-Napolitano law on immigration in 1998 (Law 40/1998) makes for the first time a specific mention of cultural mediators (Article 36 6 b: *mediatori culturali qualificati*). Article 40 states that cultural mediators (explicitly foreigners) should be used by public administrations to facilitate relations between service providers and foreigners from different ethnic, national, linguistic and religious groups, and that these cultural mediators would be provided by third-sector organizations (Merlini 2009: 59 in Amato and Garwood 2011). This led to the "Guidelines for the Recognition of the Professional Figure of Intercultural Mediators," produced by the Ministry of the Interior's Institutional Working Group for the Promotion of Intercultural Mediation, published on 21 December 2009 (Ministero dell'Interno 2009);
5 PhD dissertations: More dissertations are now focusing on public service interpreters, healthcare interpreters and the role of interpreters in this setting (e.g. Aguilar Solano 2012; Bao-Rozée 2016). There is also increasing interest on HI as a topic for master's and honors theses;
6 Academic and professional conferences on healthcare/medical interpreting: For example, the California Healthcare Interpreting Association held its 18th Annual Educational Conference in Irvine, California, on 2 March 2018 (CHIA 2018).

In addition, in 2009 a publication resulting from a research workshop held in Tel Aviv (funded by the Spencer Foundation) conducted on interpreters' and translators' identity, status and professionalization problematized the following issues about translators and interpreters: self-perception and perception of others about translators and interpreters as an occupational or a professional group (Sela-Sheffy and Shlesinger 2008). There are several differences between a profession and an occupation. An occupation refers to an activity performed for monetary compensation, while a profession refers to vocation that is associated with obtaining a higher education degree or a set of highly specialized skills. Unlike an occupation, a profession has a code of ethics and is usually regulated by a professional body statute. While a person in an occupational job gets paid for what the person produces, a professional gets paid for their expertise and skills and, generally, a professional is better paid. All professions enjoy power, and professions have a higher social power than occupations.

Remuneration is generally associated with social power, prestige and status. While the remuneration for healthcare interpreters may vary widely across countries and over time, one thing remains constant (as discussed above): compared to interpreters working in other settings (e.g. conferences, courts), remuneration for healthcare interpreters was (and is) lower. According to www.payscale.com, medical interpreters report an average of USD 20 per hour of work. Certainly this amount does not reflect the complexity of the task. The complexity of healthcare interpreting has been thoroughly documented (cf. Angelelli 2004, 2010a, 2012; Angelelli and Geist-Martin 2005; Bolden 2000; Cambridge 1999; Davidson 1998, 2000, 2001; Baraldi and Gavioli 2012; Kaufert and Putsch 1997; Metzger 1999; Meyer 2012; Prince 1986; Wadensjö 1995, 1998). Perhaps the low remuneration is connected to the perceived fragmentation of the profession, lack of standardization or the fact that healthcare interpreting still does not require a higher education degree or that there is no universally accepted validation of credentials required to enter/practice the profession.

When discussing professionalism and meeting communicative needs to access healthcare, the issue of education (see above), which lies at the basis of any profession, has been almost overlooked. This has contributed to the chicken-and-egg situation discussed above. While understandable, it has not helped the field gain the recognition it needs and deserves.

Perhaps the low remuneration may also relate to the laws of economics: it is difficult to imagine professional recognition (and thus, adequate monetary rewards) without formal education.

> A profession cannot be characterized as such without an education. Confusing training with education, encouraging interpreters to demand professional fees without offering them access to educational opportunities, or taking a leap to certification without educating for the intricacies of the field may result in putting the cart before the horse.
>
> (Angelelli 2005: 37)

B. Research, observe and reflect

Exercise 1: healthcare settings and languages

As you read this introductory chapter, you may find yourself hosting a family member/friend who does not speak the societal language of the area where you live. Or you may be traveling, accompanying a friend/relative to access healthcare across borders (e.g. for a scheduled dental treatment or cosmetic surgery) or in an emergency situation while traveling as a result of which you, your friend/

acquaintance or family member may have to access healthcare in a language in which none of you is able to communicate efficiently. As a consequence, neither you nor your family member or friend is able to participate fully in making an informed decision regarding, for example, procedure, treatment and so forth.

If none of these situations is feasible for you, go to a local clinic or hospital where they have healthcare interpreters working, explain you are interested in pursuing this career and ask if you can shadow one of the interpreters. If possible (considering privacy issues, etc.), participate or observe planned appointments related to this or a similar issue. Take notes of the context and the situation: look around and see if there are signs in the office/hospital. If there are any, in what language are they? Do these languages reflect the languages of the population living in the area? Do you understand more than one? If so, are you able to assess the appropriateness of the language used? (Do not focus only in grammar or spelling, but also pay attention to register, that is, the formal or informal way of addressing the reader.) During the encounter, try to note who speaks which language to whom and in what situation. Is there an interpreter present? If there is one, is that person a professional interpreter? A cultural mediator? A bilingual staff member asked to act as an interpreter? If there is not an interpreter present, is there one acting remotely? If no interpreter is present, how is the communication brokered? Observe the behaviors of the monolingual and the bilingual parties to the encounter and reflect upon those. At the end of the encounter, take some time to familiarize yourself with the language services/provision offered (if any) in the institution you observed. Are they delivered by professional interpreters? By bilingual hospital employees who are called upon to broker communication (e.g. bilingual receptionists, janitors, lab technicians, nurses)? What languages are covered? Is interpreting (if offered) done face-to-face or remotely (e.g. via telephone or videoconferencing)? What is the waiting time to get an interpreter? Who pays for the interpreting services? Are patients told they need to bring someone along with them who can interpret for them?

As a follow-up, research the language policy of both the organization in which the encounter you observed took place and the geographical area in which the organization is located. Is there a societal language in this area? What is it? What are the biggest linguistic minorities in this area? Are there any language provision arrangements for these minority languages? Is language provision mandated by law? Who provides language services? Individuals? Companies? If the former, are these bilingual employees of the organization? If so, is their language proficiency in the non-societal language tested? Is it taken at face value? If language services are provided by a company, what does the contract look like? Who deals with the company? Is there a language service management on site? Is interpreting booked for face-to-face or remote provision? Is it for a fixed number of hours/days in a week? What does the organization know about the qualifications/credentials of the individuals sent to interpret by the company? Think of other questions you may want to ask and research.

Once you get answers to the questions above, reflect upon the answers. What does it mean for a person who does not speak the societal language to fully participate in their own decision-making process related to a healthcare matter? What does it mean not to be able to fully participate? What are the consequences of both possibilities? Bear all of this in mind for your journal writing.

Exercise 2: the case of the Syrian refugees

As persons interested in language interpreting and intercultural communication, healthcare interpreters follow news on linguistic minorities' access to services. You may have followed the news in recent years on the displacement of Syrian refugees and the issues encountered with communication. As we discussed above, a person can become a member of a linguistic minority as an individual or as a group. The Syrian refugees are a case of a large linguistic minority group being displaced and seeking refuge in various parts of the world. Think about what happens to a group when they become displaced. Do group dynamics change? If within the group one person has little or no access to the host country language and another knows a little more, do they help each other? If the one that knows a little more is a child and the one that does not know anything is an adult, does the child help the adult? If this happens, do roles reverse? The case of the Syrian refugees put on center stage the Syrian language and the Arabic language and its different varieties. Even if these are not languages familiar to you, you can make parallels with other languages you know are used in the geographical area in which you live to analyze the situation.

Then go to www.cbc.ca/news/canada/new-brunswick/syrians-ymca-saint-john-translators-1.4440550 (last accessed June 20, 2018) and read the brief article titled "Newcomers Say Quality of Interpreting Service Provided by YMCA Is Inadequate, Especially for Doctor Visits," written by Matthew Bingley. It depicts the frustration of Syrian refugees in Canada who are facing issues with cross-linguistic/cultural communication in the host country. Syrian refugees began arriving in the Saint John area in Canada over two years ago, and since then it has been a constant struggle for them to communicate about their pains and health. The article discusses some examples in reference to accessing health services given the quality of the language translators/interpreters. Of particular interest to our discussion is the comment on not having enough reliable interpreting services to cope with medical appointments and how the poor quality/reliability of interpreting services poses a serious problem to the health and well-being of refugees. Read the segments of the article in the box below. Then follow some of the reflecting questions, make notes and get ready for your first journal entry (section D).

> Speaking through an interpreter, Mohammad Khawdam said refugees primarily use interpreters for medical visits. "A lot of people here, they don't speak very good English, and they've been at the hospital translating for people," Khawdam said. Newcomers rely on interpreters primarily for medical visits but say they often aren't up to the task. Ali Abed said

> interpreters have been so unhelpful, he has taken his complaints directly to the YMCA's administration, but did not get results.
>
> Angelique Simpson, the vice-president of newcomer and community connections, said interpreting services remain one of the YMCA's biggest challenges. The problem, she said, is a lack of Arabic speakers in the region. "We are in a constant process of trying to recruit community volunteers to help us as best as possible," she said. . . . Majad Khalit said he used to work with the YMCA as an interpreter, often working full-time hours. He needed to abandon the position for financial reasons. "How do you expect people to come and work for the YMCA when you don't want to pay anything?"
>
> The Syrian newcomers shared a story about a woman who had major issues getting a female interpreter so was sent to a hospital appointment with a male interpreter instead. When she said she couldn't be alone with the interpreter without a hijab, he allegedly grew frustrated with her and threw a pen and medical form at her back.
>
> Simpson said she couldn't comment on individual cases but was aware of what happened. "It has been brought to my attention and we are addressing it," she said. Because of time constraints, the YMCA won't always be able to provide a female interpreter when needed, Simpson said. She also said the YMCA has notified health-care providers to tell them they will have to do more to assist with interpretation in the new year.
>
> (Mathew Bingley/CBC 2018)

This article helps us reflect on population mobility, patient mobility and educational programs in language interpreting. It allows us to review the opportunities for interpreters to pursue an education in non-societal languages in general and in medical interpreting in particular. Think about what it means to face a crisis of the magnitude of the Syrian refugees and to have personal/family health issues requiring immediate attention. Is this feasible with volunteers and people who help when they can because they cannot make a living from this activity or because they are not qualified to do it professionally? As you reflect, it is helpful to differentiate on the concepts of emergency and crisis as they relate to language provision. What are your thoughts on this article and the language access situation it depicts? Reflect on the tension of supply and demand of qualified interpreters. Reflect also on the tension of educational opportunities offered in various language combinations or across languages and then compare and contrast with job opportunities available for graduates.

Search for similar articles/news segments about issues around language and access to services, and communication among other linguistic minorities in other areas.

C. Journal writing

Entry 1: Based on the activities in section B, take a few minutes to reflect on what you have observed and read. Make further notes. These personal notes will help you understand better the context in which healthcare interpreting is happening. You might compare what you have seen or experienced in your community to the situation in a different part of the world.

Entry 2: Based on what you have read, compare healthcare education/training in your country to that of an area of the world you can research. What do you see as salient differences or similarities?

Entry 3: In this chapter we have discussed how healthcare interpreting (and interpreting in general) is a complex field with many possibilities and many angles. Patients are diverse and their life circumstances are all different. They may be traveling and in need of healthcare while they are away from home, or they may be settled in a country/region where they are a linguistic minority. Regional, national and international laws also vary in how they consider access to language. In some countries, language is not a category to be protected; in others it is required to give language services to patients who cannot access healthcare without it. In some countries healthcare interpreting is funded by the government; in others it is not. Therefore, based on all of the information you have read and continue to read on this topic, draw a continuum of healthcare interpreting provision. Consider it from the perspective of the patient, the provider, the regional legal mandates and the economic resources.

D. Further tasks

- Find out if there is an association related to healthcare/medical/community interpreting in your region. It can be a local, regional, provincial/state, national or international association. Ask about membership dues and services offered to members. Is there a website you can visit? Do they have a LISTSERV service? Ask about language combinations. If you are interested, think of joining.
- If there is a professional association in your area, you may want to also familiarize yourself with the administration of the organization. Ask how it is run, if there is a board, a president and a vice president, an advisory board and so forth. Ask about qualifications held by board members; what credentials they have, or if there is a minimum requirement in terms of education in general and of healthcare/medical/community interpreting in particular. Think about how you can contribute to it.
- Do a web search using terms such as medical interpreting, healthcare interpreting and mental health interpreting; note what the search yields. Notice if you get advertisement from companies, articles to read, courses or webinars offered, blogs and so forth. Read critically the entries and materials that result from your search. Think, for example, about accuracy of information, how these entries portray or discuss healthcare interpreting. Can you differentiate between official sites of universities or institutes and those that are for commercial purposes? See if you can discriminate between goals: Is attention paid to the issue of communication, to the need for quality to give access to services, or to sell a product/service?

- Access a healthcare/medical interpreting association website and get familiar with its content. If you have accessed to some information about a training session, see the information about the trainers' expertise and teaching background and their experience in the practice of interpreting. Ask yourself if the session will give you principles and skills derived from interpreting pedagogy or examples drawn from personal experience or both.
- Do a web search to find a code of ethics for healthcare/medical interpreters and another search for a code of ethics for conference interpreters and compare. Note the similarities and the differences between both professional documents.

Notes

1 The focus of this book is on services related to healthcare and health education.
2 Conférence Internationale Permanente d'Instituts Universitaires de Traducteurs et Interprètes (International Standing Conference of University Institutes of Translators and Interpreters). See the CIUTI website at www.ciuti.org/.

References

Aguilar Solano, M. A. (2012). Positioning of volunteer interpreters in the field of public service interpreting in Spanish hospitals: A Bourdieusian perspective. Available at www.research.manchester.ac.uk/portal/files/54519703/

AIIC. (2018). *Languages taught*. Available at https://aiic.net/directories/schools/languages/ (Last Accessed April 29, 2018).

Amato, A., & Garwood, C. (2011). Cultural mediators in Italy: A new breed of linguists. *Intralinea* 13. Available at www.intralinea.org/archive/article/Cultural_mediators_in_Italy_a_new_breed_of_linguists#n15

Angelelli, C. V. (2015). *A study on public service translation in cross-border healthcare technical report*. Luxembourg: Publications Office of the European Union. ISBN 978-92-79-47163-6.

——— (2014). Interpreting in the healthcare setting: Access in cross-linguistic communication. In H. Hamilton & S. Chou (Eds.), *The Routledge handbook of language and health communication* (pp. 573–585). London and New York: Routledge.

———. (2012). Challenges in interpreters' coordination of the construction of pain. In C. Baraldi & L. Gavioli (Eds.), *Coordinating participation in dialogue interpreting* (pp. 251–268). Amsterdam and Philadelphia: John Benjamins Publishing Company.

———. (2010a). *A glimpse into the socialization of bilingual youngsters as interpreters: The case of Latino bilinguals brokering communication for their families and immediate communities*. MonTI Monografías de Traducción e Interpretación.

———. (2010b). A professional ideology in the making: Bilingual youngsters interpreting for their communities and the notion of (no) choice. *TIS Translation and Interpreting Studies* (A Publication of the American Translation and Interpreting Studies Association), *5*(1), 94–108.

______. (2007). Accommodating the need for medical interpreters: The California Endowment Interpreter Testing Project (This work was made possible by The California Endowment Grant G00005318). *The Translator*, 13(1), 63–82.

———. (2005). Healthcare interpreting education: Are we putting the cart before the horse? *The ATA Chronicle* (A Publication of the American Translators Association), *34*(11), 33–38, 55.

———. (2004). *Medical interpreting and cross-cultural communications*. Cambridge: Cambridge University Press.

———. (2000). Interpreting as a communicative event: A look through Hymes' lenses. *Meta*, *45*(4), 580–592.

Angelelli, C., & Geist-Martin, P. (2005). Enhancing culturally competent health communication: Constructing understanding between providers and culturally diverse patients. In E. B. Ray (Ed.), *Health communication in practice a case study approach* (Chapter 22, pp. 271–284). NJ: Lawrence Erlbaum Associates.

Bao-Rozée, J. (2016, May). *Using multimodal analysis to investigate the role of the interpreter*. PhD thesis, Division of Literature and Languages School of Arts and Humanities University of Stirling, United Kingdom.

Baraldi, C., & Gavioli, L. (2017). Intercultural mediation and "(non)professional" interpreting in Italian healthcare institutions. In R. Antonini, L. Cirillo, L. Rossato, & I. Torresi (Eds.), *Non-professional interpreting and translation: State of the art and future of an emerging field of research* (pp. 83–106). Amsterdam and Philadelphia: John Benjamins Publishing Company.

——— (Eds.). (2012). *Coordinating participation in dialogue interpreting*. Amsterdam and Philadelphia: John Benjamins Publishing Company.

Bingley, M. (2017, December 8). Newcomers say quality of interpreting service provided by YMCA is inadequate, especially for doctor visits. *CBC News*. Posted: 7:25 PM. (Last accessed March 2, 2018).

Bolden, G. (2000). Toward understanding practices of medical interpreting: Interpreters' involvement in history taking. *Discourse Studies*, *2*, 387–419.

British Sign Language (Scotland) Act. (2015). Asp 11. Available at www.legislation.gov.uk/asp/2015/11/contents/enacted (Last accessed March 3, 2018).

Cambridge, J. (1999). Information loss in bilingual medical interviews through an untrained interpreter. *Translator*, *5*, 201–219.

CBC News. (2017, December 8). Syrian refugees slam interpreting services in Saint John. Available at www.cbc.ca/news/canada/new-brunswick/syrians-ymca-saint-john-translators-1.4440550

CHIA. (2018). 18th Annual Educational Conference of the California Healthcare Interpreting Association, 2–3 March. Irvine, Orange County, CA.

CIUTI. Available at www.ciuti.org/about-us/profile/ (Last accessed March 4, 2018).

Council of Europe. (2001). *Common European framework of reference for languages: Learning, teaching, assessment* (CEFR). Cambridge: Cambridge University Press. Available at www.coe.int/lang-CEFR. Linguistic and Cultural Mediation. www.coe.int/en/web/lang-migrants/linguistic-and-cultural-mediation (Last accessed 23 April, 2018).

Crezee, I.H.M. (2013). *Introduction to healthcare for interpreters and translators*. Amsterdam: John Benjamins.

Davidson, B. (2001). Questions in cross-linguistic medical encounters: The role of the hospital interpreter. *Anthropological Quarterly*, *74*(4), 170–178.

———. (2000). The interpreter as institutional gatekeeper: The social-linguistic role of interpreters in Spanish-English medical discourse. *Journal of Sociolinguistics*, *4*(3), 379–405.

———. (1998). *Interpreting medical discourse: A study of cross-linguistic communication in the hospital clinic* (unpublished doctoral dissertation). Stanford University, Stanford, CA.

Drew, P., & Heritage, J. (Eds.). (1992). *Talk at work: Interaction in institutional settings*. Cambridge: Cambridge University Press.

Evrin, F., & Meyer, B. (Eds.). (2016). Non-professional interpreting and translation: Translational cultures in focus. *European Journal of Applied Linguistics Special Issue*, *4*(1).

Hilfinger Messias, DeAnne K., McDowell, L. MDiv, & Estrada, R.D. (2009, April–June). Language interpreting as social justice work: Perspectives of formal and informal healthcare interpreters. *Advances in Nursing Science*, *32*(2), 128–143. doi:10.1097/ANS.0b013e3181a3af97

Hlavac, J. (2011). Sociolinguistic profiles of users and providers of lay and professional interpreting services: The experiences of a recently-arrived Iraqi language community in Melbourne. *Translation & Interpreting*, *3*(2), 1–32.

ISO. (13611: 2014). *Interpreting: Guidelines for community interpreting*. Available at www.iso.org/standard/54082.html

Kaufert, J., & Putsch, R. (1997). Communication through interpreters in healthcare: Ethical dilemmas arising from differences in class, culture, language and power. *The Journal of Clinical Ethics*, *8*(1), 71–87.

Kennen, E. (2005). Health interpreting and health applied linguistics program creating master interpreters: Se habla español? *The Hispanic Outlook in Higher Education*, *15*(18), 30–32.

Merlini, R. (2009). Seeking asylum and seeking identity in a mediated encounter. *Interpreting*, *18*(1), 57–92.

Metzger, M. (1999). *Sign language interpreting: Deconstructing the myth of neutrality*. Washington, DC: Gallaudet University Press.

Meyer, B. (2012). Ad-hoc interpreting for partially language-proficient patients: Participation in multilingual constellations. In C. Baraldi & L. Gavioli (Eds.), *Coordinating participation in dialogue interpreting*. Amsterdam and Philadelphia: John Benjamins Publishing Company.

Mikkelson, H. (1996). Community interpreting: An emerging profession. *Interpreting*, *1*(1), 125–131.

———. (1999). *Court interpreting at a crossroads*. Available at www.acebo.com/papers/CROSSR.HTM (Last accessed April 2018).

Ministero dell'Interno. (2009). Linee di indirizzo per il riconoscimento della figura professionale del mediatore interculturale. Gruppo di Lavoro Istituzionale per la Promozione della Mediazione Interculturale. Available at www.interno.it/mininterno/export/sites/default/it/assets/files/18/00937_linee_indirizzo_mediatore_interculturale.pdf

Moreno, G., & Morales, L. S. (2010). Hablamos Juntos (together we speak). *Journal of General Internal Medicine*, *25*(12), 1282–1288.

Price, J. (1975, December 1). Foreign language interpreting in psychiatric practice. *Australia and New Zealand Journal of Psychiatric*, *9*(4), 263–267. https://doi.org/10.3109/00048677509159860

Prince, C. (1986). *Hablando con el doctor: Communication problems between doctors and their Spanish-speaking patients*. Ph.D. diss., Stanford University, Stanford, CA.

Sela-Sheffy, R., & Shlesinger, M. (2008). Strategies of image-making and status advancement of translators and interpreters as a marginal occupational group. In A. Pym, M. Shlesinger, & D. Simeoni (Eds.), *Beyond descriptive translation studies: Investigations in Homage to Gideon Toury* (pp. 79–90). Amsterdam and Philadelphia: John Benjamins.

Wadensjö, C. (1998). *Interpreting as interaction*. New York: Addison Wesley Longman Inc.

———. (1995). Dialogue interpreting and the distribution of responsibility. *Hermes, Journal of Linguistics*, *14*, 111–129.

Woloshin, S., Bickell, N. A., Schwartz, L. M., Gany, F., & Welch, H. G. (1995). Language barriers in medicine in the United States. *JAMA*, *273*(9), 724–728. doi:10.1001/jama.1995.03520330054037

Further readings

Angelelli, C. V. (2014). Interpreting in the healthcare setting: Access in cross-linguistic communication. In H. Hamilton & S. Chou (Eds.), *The Routledge handbook of language and health communication* (pp. 573–585). London and New York: Routledge.

———. (2006). Designing curriculum for healthcare interpreting education: A principles approach. In C. B. Roy (Ed.), *New approaches to interpreter education* (pp. 23–45). Gallaudet University Press.

Bibiana Clavijo, S. (2009). Formación para la profesionalización [Training for professionalization]. In various authors, *Pedagogía y didáctica de la traducción 1*, *2*(1), 67–72.

Cordero, A. (1994). The role of the university in the professionalization of the translator. In D. L. Hammond (Ed.), *Professional issues for translators and interpreters* (pp. 171–179). Amsterdam and Philadelphia: John Benjamins Publishing Company.

D'Hayer, D. (2013). Public service interpreter education: A multidimensional approach aiming at building a community of learners and professionals. In C. Schäffner, K. Kredens, & Y. Fowler (Eds.), *Interpreting in a changing landscape: Selected papers from Critical Link 6* (pp. 321–338). John Benjamins Publishing Company.

Furmanek, O. (2012). Professionalization of interpreters. In C. A. Chapelle (Ed.), *The encyclopedia of applied linguistics*. Wiley.

Pöchhacker, F., & Shlesinger, M. (Eds.). (2007). *Healthcare interpreting: Discourse and interaction*. Amsterdam and Philadelphia: John Benjamins, viii + 155 pp.

Ruiz Rosendo, L., & Conniff, D. (2015). Legislation as backdrop for the professionalisation and training of the healthcare interpreter in the United States. In JoSTrans, *The Journal of Specialized Translation* (23), 292–315.

Schäffner, C, Kredens, K., & Fowler, Y. *Interpreting in a changing landscape: Selected papers from Critical Link 6*. John Benjamins Publishing Company.

Swabey, L., & Malcolm, K. (2012). *In our hands: Educating healthcare interpreters* Washington, DC: Gallaudet University Press, 272.

Tyulenev, S., Zheng, B., & Johnson, P. (2017). A comparative study of translation or interpreting as a profession in Russia, China and Spain. In S. Tyulenev & B. Zheng (Eds.), *Toward Comparative Translation and Interpreting Studies*, *12*(2), 332–354.

Zimányi, K. (2010). The professionalisation of mental health interpreting in Ireland: Current practice. In M. Phelan & K. Zimányi (Eds.), *Community Interpreting in Ireland and Abroad*, *18*(2), 57–74.

2 Understanding the healthcare setting and its language provision policy

GOALS

In this chapter we will:

- Familiarize ourselves with the structures, cultures and stakeholders of healthcare settings.
- Learn about rights and access to language provision in healthcare settings.

LEARNING OUTCOMES

By successfully completing this chapter, readers will be able to:

- Understand the structures of a healthcare setting in general.
- Identify the stakeholders of a healthcare organization.
- Become familiar with the cultures of each of the stakeholders participating in interpreter-mediated communication in a healthcare organization.
- Connect healthcare interpreting to patients' rights and health-related legislation, especially as it pertains to issues of equality and access to information.

A. Introduction to healthcare organizations

Hospitals, clinics and community health centers are organizations embedded in specific societies. They vary in size (a clinic is generally smaller than a hospital), goals (well-being, preventive medicine, etc.), population served (e.g. a hospital specializing in children, a community center focusing on the needs of an underserved sector of the population), specializations (cancer, skin, plastic surgery) or scope (e.g. a hospital is a healthcare organization providing treatment with specialized medical and nursing staff to patients, and uses the appropriate equipment and technology to do so). Additionally, each healthcare organization has its own culture as well as its own set of rules and regulations, and adheres to regional/national and societal rules and regulations. So various layers of cultures, rules and regulations are found in healthcare settings in which healthcare interpreters

(HIs) may work. While healthcare settings share ways of doing business with other, similar organizations (e.g. healthcare organizations and government offices or business companies may share a genuine concern about health and well-being of their employees), they also have their own based on their missions. Reading the healthcare organization's mission helps to identify the healthcare values, "to inspire hope and contribute to health and well-being by providing the best care to every patient through integrated clinical practice, education, and research" (Pruthi et al. 2015: 186).

In addition to the organization specific mission and values, each of the professional groups that contributes to the healthcare organization (e.g. accountants, interpreters, lab technicians, lawyers, managers, nurses, physicians) may have their own professional standards and code of ethics by which they also abide. Thus a healthcare interpreter working in a healthcare organization juggles various cultures, rules and regulations and needs to become familiar with all of them. If the HI has been immersed in another medical culture in the past, either because they worked in a healthcare setting in other capacities (e.g. receptionist, lab technician) or because they come from a different country where they worked in a healthcare setting, the culture of the healthcare institution may or may not be similar to the healthcare interpreter's previous work environment. Perhaps the healthcare interpreter worked in a hospital in a different country, region, or with a more or less diverse patient population. Therefore, the healthcare interpreter may recognize that while there are areas of shared culture among healthcare organizations across countries/regions, there is an important part of the organizational culture that is context dependent. We now turn our attention to the importance of the context of a healthcare setting and to the factors influencing it.

Healthcare organizations: contexts and cultures

Healthcare organizations do not exist in isolation. They are part of a society and therefore permeable to the mandates of the society in which they exist. They also exist in a context. They are situated within a larger context of healthcare systems, rules and regulations. The context of an organization refers to the physical setting in which the healthcare organization sits and everything in it (Gee 2011) and any shared knowledge involved in it (e.g. organizational culture). Factors such as source of funding/income, geographical location, population served, areas of specialty and so forth contextualize what occurs within the organization. These factors influence, among other things, a healthcare organization's culture and rules in relation to language service provision. If a healthcare organization receives funding from the government or if it does not; if it is entirely public or private, national or international; if it is a healthcare organization with many branches in a country, or a more exclusive type also called a boutique hospital (McGraw-Hill Companies 2002); if it lies in a border area between two countries or two regions; if it is in an urban or rural area; or if it serves a more diverse or less diverse population – all of these factors probably influence language service provision in the organization.

As practices and expectations regarding language provision differ across healthcare systems, contexts and societies, one cannot assume that the experience from one area or one type of healthcare organization can be automatically transferred to another. Different sets of local/regional/national policies or different transpositions of macro-type policies to national ones (e.g. Directive 2011, Access to Cross-Border Healthcare in the EU and its transposition to the 28 member states of the EU at a national/regional level), impact levels and types of language provision. Thus the implementation of a general policy regarding language provision/access to language services on the part of individuals who do not share the societal language is not universal and may not transfer from country to country or state to state. The issue of (not) paying much attention to language or communication across languages and cultures seems to be a persistent one in healthcare organizations. The same holds true for pondering the linguistic and cultural differences in more innovative ways instead of considering them a problem. Linguistic and cultural differences are facts of life in our diverse world. The problem is refusing to acknowledge these facts. Multiple solutions exist to bridge them and they are not costly. In fact, many times, catering to a diverse patient population opens different markets or possibilities (Angelelli 2015), and many medical associations are taking advantage of the new trend. In some geographic areas or for some sectors of the population, language access and intercultural/linguistic communication appear to continue to be either disregarded or, what may be even worse, dealt with using homemade solutions, some of which may have fatal consequences.

In addition to a distinct context, each healthcare organization, like any other organization, has its own culture (Davies et al. 2000). It is important to learn the healthcare organization's culture because it permeates every aspect of daily work. When staff members join a healthcare organization, they may be introduced to its culture directly or indirectly in various ways, from simple statements such as "it is how we do stuff around here" (Robinson and Tyndale-Biscoe 2012) or "it is our way of doing things" (Angelelli 2004) to more elaborate statements that include detailed descriptions of the healthcare organization vision, mission, values, beliefs and so forth (e.g. Pruthi et al. 2015). These descriptions may or may not include statements on patient-centered care or patients' full participation in decision-making about care, to give just two examples. When a healthcare organization values linguistic and cultural diversity, one would expect to find some affirmation of this valorization embedded in the mission/vision. This would be a good start, although it does not necessarily end there. One then needs to look for evidence of how the healthcare organization actually materializes support for users of non-societal languages so that they can access healthcare services. Healthcare interpreters need to be aware of the healthcare organization's recognition and valorization of language diversity in their places of work.

Research on healthcare organization culture is conducted for various purposes: to understand or measure employees' perceptions of a hospital culture (e.g. Robinson and Tyndale-Biscoe 2012), to determine if employee's perceptions are associated with hospital performance (e.g. Zhou et al. 2011) and to explore the relationship between organization culture and quality of healthcare (Davies et al.

2000). Interestingly, in the literature on healthcare organization culture and values (e.g. Andrulis and Brach 2007; Davies et al. 2000; Pruthi et al. 2015; Robinson and Tyndale-Biscoe 2012), statements on language provision to facilitate access to healthcare services when patients belong to a different linguistic group do not abound. This is problematic, especially on the part of international healthcare organizations, because medical tourism and patient mobility are on the rise.

The culture of a healthcare organization, its conceptualization of communication and the rules and regulations by which it abides may vary widely from area to area and organization to organization. Healthcare interpreters need to familiarize themselves with these variations. Understanding differences across settings and organizations and becoming familiar with the medical setting or the healthcare organizations in which one works are important for all stakeholders. It is as important for language services providers (e.g. interpreters, translators and mediators, whether they are freelance individuals or part of an agency/company) as it is for healthcare providers, as well as for patients and family members. And because stakeholders are a key part of the organization in which one works, we now turn our attention to the players that healthcare interpreters may come across in their daily work.

Stakeholders in healthcare organizations

In this section we discuss some of the stakeholders from healthcare organizations with whom healthcare interpreters may come into contact in the course of doing their work. This is important for two reasons: (1) to review some of the participants for whom they will interpret in a healthcare encounter and (2) to understand who makes decisions on language services, who determines quality and so forth. As we reflect on participants and their interactions throughout the book, in addition to the positions they hold within the organization, it is important to pay close attention to their backgrounds, social factors and ways of speaking. This is helpful to understand why they relate to each other in the way they do, whether they share the same language or they use the help of a language-service provider (e.g. an interpreter, a cultural/linguistic mediator) to communicate with others.[1]

Healthcare providers (HCPs)

Healthcare providers are key to helping the patient with the healthcare issue at hand. They have the technical knowledge and expertise the patients need. These days, due to the way some healthcare systems are set in many areas of the world, HCPs may only have limited time to interact with a patient. They may only be able to allocate 10 or 15 minutes per patient to accomplish the goal of the visit. They may even be limited to discussing one specific issue per encounter. So, much to their chagrin, providers are pressed for time and have limited interaction with patients.

Even when physicians are better educated and more scientific than ever before, these attributes do not necessarily translate in them communicating more effectively with their patients (Jacobs et al. 2001). At times, HCPs may speak in technical language ("medicalese") or in a register that is too formal for patients to understand (Angelelli 2004). Or even if they do monitor their verbal production, they may not pay too much attention to their nonverbal interactions (Lee et al. 2002). In addition, HCPs may or may not be aware of a patient's place of origin, culture, language or degree of literacy to contextualize or tailor their explanations and make them more understandable or useful for patients. The more specialized a healthcare member of staff is, or the higher up in rank, the more focused they are on the issue at hand. As a consequence, the less time the provider has available to invest in provider-patient relationship building. This may not be aligned with patients' expectations. Research studies report that some patients expect HCPs to engage in building a provider-patient relationship, and they recognize the difference when providers in other countries do take the time to do this (cf. Crookes et al. 2015). Studies in medical tourism discuss medical tourists' reports of interactions with healthcare providers working abroad. In the case of medical tourism in South America, reports indicate patients acknowledging that they would change destinations based on the courtesy and personal service they can get in some countries (e.g. Argentina) over others.

Ideally, a collaborative relationship between physician and patient is a therapeutic alliance in which doctor and patient are partners in a common struggle against an illness (Adler 2002). When patients are treated as partners in the medical dialogue instead of mere reporters of symptoms, (1) they become more willing to ask questions or express concerns and (2) they are more likely to receive useful information about their illness and therapeutic plan. In addition, HCP-patient collaboration increases the patient's autonomy, and the higher the quality of the HCP-patient relationship, the better the therapeutic outcomes. Moreover, autonomous and more informed patients can make informed decisions (Entwistle et al. 2010). The establishment of an empathic bond (Candib 1995) facilitates collaboration and constructs a positive relationship, thus reducing the likelihood of a discordant one. When providers do not speak the language of the patient, an interpreter is called in to facilitate communication. Thus, during the interpreted encounter, interpreters need to be mindful and facilitate both the communication and the provider-patient relationship.

Patients (and their family members/caregivers)

During healthcare encounters, patients are sometimes alone and sometimes accompanied by either a family member, a friend, or a caregiver. Family members may be more or less involved in the management of the patient's healthcare in general and, consequently, more or less informed on the issue at hand. Caregivers or friends may also participate in an encounter when family members cannot be available. In some cultures, HCPs prefer to discuss issues with the patient and the family/friends/caregivers. They report that questions are asked of family members to triangulate with what patients are reporting (Angelelli 2015: 14). The participation of family members is essential to make decisions, because in some cultures, decisions are not made exclusively by the patient, but by the family. This is the case in more community-oriented cultures. These orientations also show different conceptualizations of confidentiality and privacy.

Most patients want as much information as possible from their HCPs. HCPs need to offer this information in a manner that is useful and understandable to the patients. Sometimes, HCPs may underestimate the type and amount of information a patient can handle (Berwick 2009). Whereas healthcare HCPs from countries in northwestern Europe and North America are depicted as focusing more on the patient or the patient's proxy holder as a result of following a patient-oriented approach (Crezee 2013), efforts have been made on the part of providers to change paradigms. For example, a patient-centered model began to be implemented in 2006 (American Hospital Association and Institute for Family-Centered Care Resource Guide 2006; Johnson et al. 2008). This model "included the patient and family member participation in medical rounds, patient decision making on food and clothing (as allowed by health status) and patient ownership of medical records with clinicians needing to have permission to gain access to them" (Berwick 2009: 561).

When patients do not share the language of providers, healthcare interpreters are called to broker their communication. Healthcare interpreters should be mindful of how patients may perceive them, their work and their role. Because patients may consider interpreters their concordant or emphatic interlocutor, patients may turn to interpreters for clarification, examples, among others. Providing useful and understandable information is the responsibility of providers, and patients need to be reminded of this.

Administrative staff

The administrative staff plays a key role in the running of the organization, from the everyday tasks to the strategic planning for new developments and so forth. In some larger hospitals in which we find a language service unit, it is not unusual to see translators or interpreters in managerial positions running these units on the basis of their technical (as opposed to managerial) knowledge. In addition to the daily management of the unit and the workloads of the employees, part of their responsibilities may include the design of curriculum for professional development of HCPs and hospital administrators (specific courses on linguistically and culturally diverse patients, how to work with interpreters, how to establish teamwork with interpreters/translators, etc.). If the hospital does not have in-house interpreting staff or an in-house language service unit, it is the administrative staff who generally are in charge of organizing language provision (through contacting freelancers, agencies, etc.). Administrative staff vary in their understanding and conceptualization of the work of interpreters (and translators). Healthcare interpreters need to be aware of issues that may arise and be ready to engage in educating others about the intricacies of the job.

Providers of language services

Providers of language services are key to enabling HCPs and patients to communicate when they do not share a language. Whether acting as interpreters, translators or linguistic (sometimes called language) or cultural mediators, providers of language services generally have an understanding of the patient's place of origin, culture and language background. This does not mean, however, that interpreters, translators or language/cultural mediators are experts either in the culture of the patient or in the language variety the patient uses. For example, among the 22+ Spanish-speaking countries/areas of the world, there are important variations in pragmatics (e.g. how politeness is expressed) and vocabulary (e.g. how they say "flu"), the structure of the language (some Spanish-speaking countries/areas use different subject pronouns such as *tú* or *vos*; in some French-speaking countries/areas, speakers may use the verb *savoir* instead of *pouvoir*) or paralinguistic elements of language such as gesture or body language. Professional healthcare interpreters know the limits of their knowledge and they know how to seek clarification of issues rather than making assumptions about them. They therefore are in a position to tailor their own ways of speaking and make them understandable to the patient and the HCP.

There are several differences among interpreters, translators and language or cultural mediators. Healthcare interpreters (who are at the center of this book) are covered below. Translators should not be confused with interpreters. While interpreting involves the communication of oral or signed messages in real time, translation involves the communication of a written/video/electronic message into another language in written/video/electronic form and a certain period of time is allocated for the task. In addition to the difference between written and oral/signed form and the time constraints, interpreting conceptualizes communication as the result of human interaction. As such, interpreting means brokering both the content and meaning of messages. Meaning, as stated above, is more than words. It encompasses body language, facial expressions and gestures, intonation contours and other paralinguistic features used during an interpreted communicative event. Interpreting may occur across a wide range of social factors (gender, ethnicity, socio-economic class, education, age and nationality).

While translation and interpreting are professions with recognized university degrees in many parts of the world, currently there is no BA, MA or PhD in language or cultural mediation. In some countries (e.g. Italy, Spain), there are several university courses and the figure of the cultural mediator is recognized by law (Italy Law 40/1998 – Article 36 6 b). In addition, in some cases the cultural mediator is more protected than the translator/interpreter (see Chapter 1; Ministero dell'Interno 2009). In Italy, the recognition of the cultural mediator as a professional figure is further increased by the number of other names used to refer to them, from "cultural mediator" to "linguistic-cultural mediator," "intercultural animator" and "intercultural operator" (Halba 2009–21). It is also worth mentioning that the term "provider of language service" may include not only individuals but also businesses in the language industry such as translation/interpreting agencies, telephone companies offering telephone interpreting and others.

Healthcare interpreters

HIs are professionals with specific qualifications, credentials and/or a degree in interpreting or a related field. Committed to carrying out an assignment successfully, healthcare interpreters possess interpreting skills, are proficient in at least two languages (spoken or sign) and have expertise and experience working in healthcare communication. The healthcare interpreter observes the code of ethics of the profession and brokers communication between two users of different languages in real time. Healthcare interpreters work face-to-face and sometimes remotely using technology such as videoteleconference, wired or wireless phone or other intelligent portable devices. They strive to convey every semantic element (content, intention, form, gist, gesture, pauses, silences and tone) of the message. They engage in interactive types of communication, which usually means working in a dialogue form and interpreting in and out of the two languages (also known as a bi-directional and dialogic pattern). Most of the time, healthcare interpreters work consecutively. There are cases in which they may also interpret simultaneously and remotely (e.g. a doctor-patient conference with family members when not all can be on site to attend a meeting, in which a procedure needs to be explained or consent to a procedure needs to be explored). Simultaneous interpreting is also used as the main mode in hospitals which are equipped for this purpose (e.g. at California Hope), wired through regular phone lines using speakerphones. These hospitals report using simultaneous mode for two reasons: it saves time and it allows for more privacy between provider and patient (Angelelli 2004, Hornberger et al. 1996).

Ad hoc interpreters

Ad hoc interpreters do not hold a degree in interpreting, nor do they have any other qualifications or credentials. They may or may not have any experience in performing the task at hand, and may or may not observe any code of ethics. They may exhibit the ability to speak both languages needed for a task at hand and volunteer to perform the role of an interpreter. At times, rather than volunteering, they may be directed to do it by the pertaining authority (e.g. bilingual employees in hospitals may be asked to stop doing their work and assist with communication because interpreters are not available). Speakers of the non-societal language cannot always access services through interpreters, as there may be none available. Therefore, in the absence of qualified interpreters, users of non-societal languages often resort to ad hoc interpreters to communicate with speakers of societal languages. These include bilingual service providers (e.g. medical assistants, laboratory technicians, receptionists, janitors) as well as family members or friends who are asked to step in and help broker communication with various degrees of success. This may have serious consequences that undermine equal access to services. We discuss some examples in detail below.

Issues of language and access in healthcare organizations

Access to information

When we discuss access to information in general, we need to start by defining what access to healthcare information means in current times. In the past, access to healthcare information used to be mostly limited to people who were in the healthcare professions. These days, information is ready available to the general public. Current technologies allow for information on medical conditions, procedures, treatments and so forth to be distributed in different ways and it is readily accessible in various formats. This, however, does not mean the information available is always valid or reliable, or that information is readily accessible to everyone. It means that for those who (1) can afford technology, (2) know how to use it, (3) can discriminate factual information from scams, opinions, anecdotes or perceptions (4) understand how to conduct web searches, and (5) can perform web searches independently, there is indeed a vast amount of information available. And last but not least, while information can be physically accessible, it may not be accessible for readers with various degrees of literacy and education. So, we should not underestimate the value of understanding the accessible information.

Thus, when we consider access we have to consider computer literacy, age range, language background and socio-economic status that allow access to technology. Currently, while many people may enjoy instant connectivity to web-based information and social network support (or lack thereof) through myriad devices, others may rely only on their interactions with healthcare providers or younger family members to obtain the healthcare information they may need. Thus access to information can be direct and virtual, facilitated by a provider, a family member or a friend with various degrees of expertise. Access to a provider can be face-to-face or remote. It is not uncommon to call a help line and have a nurse conduct triage over the phone to determine if a patient should be seen by a provider or not.

Communication problems due to inability to access language and information are at the core of misunderstandings causing adverse events with fatal consequences. Patients who cannot access communication in the place where they are seeking care are considered higher-risk patients. Communication issues due to HCPs and patients not sharing a language delay treatment and jeopardize the trust between provider and patient. These issues can be overcome with interpreting or mediation. A high percentage of the information that goes into the diagnosis emerges from the interaction between patient and provider (Wilson 2013). Therefore, as communication between provider and patient in the same language is challenging enough, it is not surprising to hear it can be exponentially more complex across languages and cultures. Legislation and regulatory standards on language provision vary across the world, and in some areas there is none. In some countries (e.g. Australia, Belgium, Canada, Greece, Spain, United Kingdom), legislation requires that interpreting services be provided at no charge to the patient. This is not the case in all countries even within the same macro-structure (e.g. Germany). In other countries, provision depends on the type of public funding the healthcare organization has (e.g. in the United States this only applies to organizations receiving federal funding and patients whose income is below a certain threshold). In other countries there is simply no language service provision.

Language provision in healthcare organizations

In addition to complying with language access requirements and improving patients' satisfaction, incorporating interpreting services into healthcare improves patient safety and health outcomes. Interpreters need to be seen as partners in communication between providers and patients. There are different ways in which interpreting services can be delivered in a healthcare organization (face-to-face, video remote and telephone interpreting). This flexibility helps meet needs immediately and in languages that are less commonly used in the area in which the healthcare organization is located. However, in spite of accessibility, affordability and flexibility, still not all healthcare organizations provide language services (Angelelli 2015).

When healthcare organizations do offer language provision, support may be integrated in-house (as staff interpreters) or hired out (from agencies that can supply interpreters in a variety of languages). If in house, staff may be found in the form of service department within the organization (e.g. interpreting services, cultural mediation) or part of another department (e.g. patient services). When interpreters/cultural mediators are hired as staff members, they undergo an admission process as any other staff member in the organization (validating credentials, a human resources interview, etc.). In addition, they are tested specifically for the skills required in the job they are hired to perform. For interpreters/mediators, this generally means language tests on both working languages to seek evidence that the interpreter is literate in both languages, that they can perform interpreting and also that they are familiar with medical language (i.e. language for specific purposes, as the one used in a medical setting). On-site interpreters are the best choice for certain interactions that require the interpreter to be present, to assure continuity of services and development of a shared organizational culture, and to have control over quality.

Interpreters working off-site may be the best choice for remote areas or when access is complicated (e.g. due to an emergency), or for languages of limited diffusion. New technologies (e.g. video-remote conferencing equipment), software (e.g. Skype or GoToMeeting) and new applications of web-conferencing software (StarLeaf, Wire, Livestorm, Webinato) have simplified the access to remote interpreters 24 hours a day, 7 days a week. Hospitals may have contracts with agencies providing access to interpreters remotely via telephone or video conference in addition to in-house staff for the cases discussed above (Angelelli 2004) or when all on-site interpreters are busy. Videoconferences are much more affordable these days and video interpreting has emerged as the option that emulates most closely the in-person experience. The interpreter has access to gestures and visual cues. Video interpreting has always been the preferred option for sign language users. When the interpreter is not present, the provider may need to orient the interpreter to the physical context and the case.

Healthcare organizations can make informed decisions on types of systems and/or devices which may constitute the best options for the situation. In most cases, speakerphones are the best option because they provide access to more than one party at the same time. A patient, for example, may be accompanied by a family members or a friend, or the provider may be in the room with a nurse, an assistant or an intern. A speakerphone would provide everyone in the room with access to information. When healthcare organizations use speakerphones, they train their interpreters to interpret simultaneously. This has proven not only to save time but also to give providers and patients more space and privacy without the presence of an interpreter (Hornberger et al. 1996). A speakerphone, however, would pose a problem in a public area (reception room, pharmacy) if privacy is required. In these cases, dual handheld devices would provide privacy.

At present, the discussions about language provision and access cannot be limited to local patients who reside in a country/region/area. Given the increase in patient mobility triggered by medical tourism, legislation (e.g. EU Directive 2011/24/EU) or reciprocity agreements between countries/regions, discussions on intercultural/linguistic communication, access to language, informed consent to and participation in one's treatments are applicable to patients without borders. Interestingly these discussions on language and access do not abound in studies that specifically focus on medical tourism and patient mobility. For example, in the 46-chapter *Handbook on Medical Tourism and Patient Mobility*, only one chapter mentions language concordance as a determining factor for immigrants from South America or Latin America to seek healthcare in Argentina (Hadler 2015). Medical tourism, patient mobility and migration are here to stay. Therefore, in addition to the current diversity of patients observed in healthcare organizations today, delivering healthcare services beyond borders highlights the need for healthcare systems to accommodate the needs of patients with passports (Cohen 2015) using a variety of languages. Undoubtedly, this accommodation requires quality language provision such as interpreting services.

Language provision and the law: healthcare interpreting, patients' rights and health-related legislation

To understand the legal rights to language access that patients have, we turn to legislation, statutes and laws. In some countries, we find laws that specifically regulate interpreting, translation and cultural/linguistic mediation. In other countries, legislation is not as specific, as "language" or "linguistic access" may not be categories protected by law (e.g. the European Union in Angelelli 2015: viii), while in others, language may be a proxy for other categories like national origin (United States). As stated earlier, each country is different. Therefore, it behooves healthcare interpreters to be aware of their professional standing vis-à-vis the law in the areas where they work. Now we will consider some examples of legislation from different parts of the world.

AUSTRALIA

With a steady increase in population diversity, blending communicative needs resulting from migration, asylum seekers, First Peoples of Australia or Auslan users, Australia has taken many steps to provide language access to non-societal language users. This is evident by the quantity and quality of spoken and sign language services offered in most areas of the country. In addition, Australia has made efforts to incorporate cultural diversity in medical practices.

An example of this is the recent consultation administered by the Migrant and Refugee Women's Health Partnership on the Competency Standard Framework for culturally responsive clinical practice. This new framework focuses on people from migrant and refugee backgrounds, not on First Peoples. However, it acknowledges that "Aboriginal and Torres Strait Islander Peoples, as First Peoples of Australia, have a unique place in Australia's culturally diverse society." It further acknowledges that both First Peoples of Australia as well as people from migrant and refugee backgrounds have distinctly diverse starting points and face unique access challenges as they engage with both clinicians and the healthcare system more generally. In the Framework, Competency 7 discusses the collaboration between clinicians and interpreters. It presents three sub-competencies related to clinicians' recognition of the interpreter's role and responsibilities. These are:

> 7.1 Clinicians recognise the role of the interpreter in the clinical setting, their skills, their responsibilities and their scope of practice.
> 7.2 Clinicians recognise that the on-site interpreter cannot be asked to provide written translations of material, but may be asked to do a sight translation.
> 7.3 Clinicians inform interpreters on the nature of the consultation prior to its commencement where possible, recognising the need to assist the interpreter to prepare for the information that may need to be interpreted.
>
> (First Consultation Draft 2018: 15)

In addition, the Australian medical code of ethics, titled *The Good Medical Practice: A Code of Conduct for Doctors in Australia*, states that "Good communication underpins every aspect of good medical practice" (Medical Board of Australia 2014). Clinicians must ensure there is clear and effective communication in the patient-clinician relationship so that they can effectively manage the patient's healthcare. The patient needs to understand the discussion that takes place and needs to understand the proposed management and treatment.

Compared to supplying translation and interpreting services to a diverse population of refugees and immigrants, language provision for users of indigenous languages is more complex. In the Northern Territory (around the Darwin area), for example, where more than 100 languages and dialects are spoken, language provision is challenging for a user of an indigenous language who needs to access healthcare services and does not speak English. In hospitals and clinics in Katherine and Darwin, there are language-service offices or patient-services offices on site that deal with language diversity and handle requests for translation or interpreting. The Australian government offers free interpreting and translation services through the Home Office, Department of Home Affairs (www.tisnational.gov.au 2019) and Department of Social Services (www.dss.gov.au/our-responsibilities/settlement-services/programs-policy/settle-in-australia/help-with-english/free-interpreting-service 2019). Interpreting services are free for patients who are hospitalized or who have an appointment.

For those who need interpreting services and are neither patients in the hospital nor outpatients with appointment, the Northern Territory Government (NTG) also regulates the interpreting fees charged per hour for interpreting. These fees are differentiated following the National Accreditation Authority for Translators and Interpreters (NAATI) three-level classification for Australia: professional, paraprofessional and non-accredited. There is a significant difference between the rate for hiring at the interpreter level ($152 for up to two hours), the paraprofessional level ($112 for up to two hours) and the non-accredited level ($72 for up to two hours). All the information about interpreting services, booking, fees and availability is available on the NTG website only in English (Northern Territory Government 2018).

During a study examining healthcare interpreter's beliefs and attitudes toward their role (Angelelli and Slatyer 2010), surveys, field observations, focus groups and interviews were conducted in various hospitals, clinics and language-service agencies in the Northern Territory, Melbourne and Sydney. When asking for information about interpreting in indigenous languages in the Northern Territory, the manager of patient services on site explained that because it is not always possible to identify or have access to a professional interpreter for indigenous languages, agencies hold workshops to help volunteers who are speakers of some indigenous languages and have some degree of proficiency in English. These volunteers help patients communicate with English speakers and navigate the healthcare system to bridge the cultural and communicative gap. In part this is because it is not common for English-speaking interpreters to be proficient in indigenous languages. To help the supply of language interpreters between English and aboriginal languages, some agreements and opportunities are in place for indigenous language speakers who have some degree of proficiency in English and wish to pursue a career in interpreting. With funding from the Australian government, interpreting agencies and universities came together to deliver a curriculum for bilinguals with indigenous, refugee or immigrant languages. The learning opportunities (training) vary across areas from a couple of hours depending on availability of trainers to a couple of weeks. It is generally performed by local interpreters who pass their experiences on to the newcomers. Materials provided include glossaries as well as the code of ethics and scenarios for role plays. During the sessions, participants also share their experiences. Based on reports from agency managers and hospital staff working in social services or patients' services offices, it appears to be a struggle to recruit bilinguals with enough proficiency in English.

EUROPEAN UNION (EU)

In the EU, a mosaic of multilingual and multicultural societies, EU citizens exercise their right to mobility with more frequency. Mobile citizens traveling or residing in another member state (MS) from time to time need to access healthcare services where they do not (yet) speak the societal language. These patients may need different types/levels of language support in order to access safe and high-quality healthcare. The support can take various forms: (1) information in their own language; (2) translation of specific documents (e.g. medical records or documents for reimbursement); or (3) interpreting and/or cultural mediation. In the European Union both the mobility of citizens and their access to healthcare are rights guaranteed in the EU Charter. Language access and right to language are not explicitly mentioned, however.

A research project conducted on Directive 2011/24/EU entitled "A Study of Public Service Translation in Access to Cross-Border Healthcare" investigated language provision and access to healthcare across five member states: Germany, Greece, Italy, Spain and the United Kingdom (Angelelli 2015). To determine if language is a right or an enabling condition within EU law, we analyzed the four principal documents that provide the framework to regulate EU cross-border healthcare: (1) the Charter of Fundamental Rights of the European Union, which establishes the rights for citizens of the Union; (2) the Treaty on the Functioning of the European Union, which was established from the agreements of the Lisbon Treaty, and defines the mechanisms for the governance of the Union; (3) Regulation (EC) 883/2004, which establishes norms and competencies for the provision of healthcare to certain classes of cross-border patients; and (4) Directive 2011/24/EU, which intends to clarify the legal relationship between patients' rights and cross-border care (Department of Health 2012). None of these documents contemplates how EU patients may access information or communicate with healthcare staff and providers in a language that is not their own. There is only one exception that contemplates access to language in the EU: Directive 2010/64/EU for the legal field. It stipulates the right to interpreting and translation in the framework of criminal proceedings only (Official Journal of the European Union 2004, 2010, 2011).

Although it is obvious that access to information is crucial for anyone to pursue healthcare assistance in a member state, none of the four documents constituting the EU framework explicitly refers to language provision for EU citizens or legal residents in that condition. In the absence of a clear EU legislative guidance, each member state has its own legislation and those vary considerably from one member state to another. In the United Kingdom, for example, the Equality Act (2010) mandates institutions to provide language services so that patients can access healthcare services. In Germany, the only reference to language in legislation is in regard to obtaining consent from patients in a language that patients understand. Neither in Germany nor in Greece is there evidence of legislation considering the provision of language services to patients who do not speak the societal language. In both Italy and Spain, regional languages are protected by law, and consequently information to patients must be offered in these languages. In most cases there is not any legislation that guarantees comprehensive language services to patients. The absence of formal language guidance in EU legislation regarding healthcare leads to a poorer quality of healthcare for those patients who cannot access societal languages.

Another goal of the study was to identify languages services offered and what is considered best practice (Angelelli 2015: 83). Relevant to this discussion is the provision of language interpreting. Three types of interpreting provision are offered in the healthcare settings observed: face-to-face/on site, videoconference interpreting and telephone interpreting. Except for the United Kingdom, where legislation (Equality Act 2010) mandates the provision of interpreters for patients who cannot access English, only 2 percent of the settings observed (including private hospitals and clinics) engaged healthcare interpreters. Even in the UK, while the National Health Service strives to provide interpreters (as it is mandated by law) in some of the observed sites (e.g. urban accident and emergency department of a large hospital; smaller urban specialized pavilion in respiratory infections), informants (nurses, physicians, lab technicians) reported that interpreters could not be used at all times because they are very expensive. Informants also stated that as providers, they resort to drawings and signs.

In Italy, institutions frequently call upon intercultural mediators to provide language services. In Spain, regional languages are recognized and bilingual medical service is offered in those languages by medical and bilingual professionals. This includes the provision of bilingual forms and documents as well as the employment of bilingual staff and providers. For languages other than regional languages, the provision is the responsibility of each hospital. There are differences between healthcare organizations in the public and private sectors. Private sector hospitals offer translation and interpreting services in different languages for affluent medical tourists. In both Germany and Greece, professional language services are limited and were only observed in relation to consent forms and videoconference interpreting in private clinics, respectively. In the United Kingdom, public healthcare institutions routinely offer professional language services to patients who do not understand written or spoken English. These institutions have equality and diversity departments in charge of guaranteeing equal access (Angelelli 2015: 11).

At times there is unequal access to the highest level of protection that all EU citizens are guaranteed because, in the absence of formal legislation and policy guidance, organizations and patients are left to their own devices to meet communicative needs. There is no legislation in place at the EU level that defines the responsibility for who is to provide language services in the healthcare setting. Language access, the right to interpreting and translation in healthcare are not stated in EU law. Thus, because healthcare interpreters or public-service interpreters are mobile too, while working in healthcare interpreting within the EU it is important to understand the differences among member states and the regional, national and EU legislation. Healthcare organizations are bound by national or regional legislation and policy guidance.

In conclusion, language services for patients is not provided in an even and consistent manner in the EU. Very often, healthcare institutions call upon ad hoc language brokers (bilingual staff, family members, friends, volunteers) to perform translation, interpreting or language/cultural mediation without compensation since professional services are not offered. In most cases, professional language support is not provided at all because it is perceived as costly and not always essential. This calls into question the right to access safe and high-quality healthcare, as stated in Directive 2011/24/EU.

UNITED STATES

In the United States, at the federal level, the 1964 Civil Rights Act continues to be "the single most important piece of legislation for providing limited-English-proficiency individuals a legal right to language assistance services" (Chen 2004; Chen et al. 2007). With diversity increasing at a steady pace, as evidenced by the more than 200 different languages spoken in the country, there is an increased pressure on healthcare systems and clinicians to ensure equal access to services on the part of linguistic minorities. The wording of the law is as follows: "No person in the United States shall, on the ground of race, color or national origin, be excluded from participation in, be denied the benefits of, or be subjected to any discrimination under any program or activity receiving federal assistance" (US Code 1964).

The purpose of the Civil Rights Act was twofold. On the one hand, it ensured that federal money was not used to support discriminatory programs or activities. On the other hand, because language was treated as a proxy for national origin by the federal government in federally funded programs and activities, people who speak a language other than English are entitled to equal treatment as the one received by English speakers. In 1980, the Department of Health and Human Services (HHS) issued a note stating that no person should be subject to discrimination from HHS programs on the basis of having a primary language which is other than English. The HHS Office of Civil Rights (OCR) investigates complaints related to linguistic barriers. The legal responsibility to provide language access applies across all federal programs, and healthcare is no exception. This does not mean there is always compliance.

The case of 13-year-old Gricelda Zamora of California illustrates a violation of rights to language or language access in healthcare services. Like many children whose parents speak limited English, Gricelda served as her family's interpreter, and in 1999 she died as a result of no access to language. This case clearly shows that the battle for language access in healthcare in the United States is not won. The following is a brief summary of what was reported.

> When she developed severe abdominal pain, her parents took her to the hospital. Unfortunately, Gricelda was too sick to interpret for herself, and the hospital did not provide an interpreter. After a night of observation, her Spanish-speaking parents were told, without the aid of an interpreter, to bring her back immediately if her symptoms worsened, and otherwise to follow up with a doctor in three days. However, what her parents understood from the conversation was that they should wait three days to see the doctor. After two days, with Gricelda's condition deteriorating, they felt they could no longer wait, and rushed her back to the emergency department. Doctors discovered

> she had a ruptured appendix. She was airlifted to a nearby medical center in Phoenix, where she died a few hours later.
>
> (Chen et al. 2007: 362)

Cases like this are, unfortunately, not just a thing from the past. To avoid a repeat of this shocking story, the following four recommendations were made (Chen et al. 2007: 367):

1 A need for a financing mechanism for language assistance services across payers. Currently, there is a huge variation across institutions in whether (and if so, how) they provide language services to speakers of other languages. A consistent financing mechanism would minimize the current variation and bring consistency to the state. Insurers would contract with and pay medical interpreters or language agencies directly to serve their patients, rather than having the providers involved in screening, selecting and paying the interpreter.
2 A need for a significant investment in developing a qualified and professional medical interpreter workforce, in terms of increasing both the number and quality of medical interpreters. Certification, which exists in a few states (e.g. Washington, Oregon, Indiana and North Carolina) and has gained momentum in a number of others, is a critical part of assuring the quality of interpreting and would benefit from coordination and standardization across states. Currently there are three certifying bodies for medical interpreters: the National Board of Certification for Medical Interpreters (NBCMI); the Certification Commission for Healthcare Interpreters (CCHI); and the Department of Social and Health Services/Language Testing and Certification Program Washington State (DSHS/LTC). However, without appropriate remuneration for language access services in healthcare, it will continue to be difficult to attract qualified individuals into the medical interpreter workforce.
3 A need for healthcare providers to understand the harmful effects of language barriers and the benefits of working with professional medical interpreters, so that they advocate for language assistance services for their limited-English-speaking patients in the same way they would advocate for any important diagnostic test.
4 A need for limited English-speaking patients to be aware of their legal rights and take the necessary steps within their power to seek their enforcement. Limited English-speaking patients are relatively disempowered in the US healthcare system. Thus increasing patient's awareness alone has proved not to be sufficient to improve language access. Patients/family members reporting cases at the organizations in which their rights were put in jeopardy to filing Office of Civil Rights complaints has been key to improving language provision, which in turn results in better and more consistent language access through services such as interpreting and translation across the country. Filing OCR complaints continues to be an important driving force for legislative change in the United States.

The regions of the world with a more diverse stable population are in some ways the most developed in understanding and addressing the disparities in language access to healthcare and enjoy the most accessible networks for healthcare interpreting. These diverse regions are also the ones with more challenges in terms of variations in cross-linguistic/cultural communication around healthcare and well-being, given the budgetary constraints, health disparities and geographic extension. As has become evident from the examples discussed, even when healthcare is mandated by policy, it is always dependent on the balance between supply and demand to meet language provision on the one hand and appropriate funding/budget appropriation on the other.

B. Research, observe and reflect

If you live in an area in which you can access healthcare organizations, make plans to visit at least two types of the following organizations: a private specialized clinic (e.g. fertility clinic, plastic surgery); a public clinic; and a general hospital. Make an inventory of the services offered. Inquire whether (and if so, how) they accommodate patients who do not speak the societal language. Observe the signage in the healthcare organization. If you have the chance to meet an interpreter, be prepared to have a brief conversation/interview. Plan questions about the interpreters' working conditions in this organization (workload, breaks), the requirements for hiring interpreters and so forth. Find out if the organization allows family members, bilingual staff members from the hospital/clinic, or volunteers to interpret. Pay attention to the reactions, the expectations and the facial expressions of the interpreter as they answer your questions.

C. Journal writing

You probably have visited a healthcare organization (whether for your own care or to accompany or visit a friend) before reading this chapter. Think back about this visit/place. It could have been a hospital, clinic, center in your area or in another place while you were visiting/working. At the time of your visit, you probably were not thinking about the context or culture of the healthcare setting. Now, and on the basis of what you have just read, what could you say about the context of the organization you visited? Think about medical settings that you have visited and where you have been conducting observations. Write about things/issues involving diversity of culture or language which you may not have reflected on or which caught your attention.

D. Further tasks

In your area there may be more or less linguistic diversity. What do you know about languages used in your area? Do a search and look for statistics on language diversity in your region/country. If your area is diverse, focus on it. If not, focus on another country/region of the world known for its diversity. Do a search where you are based, and look into legislation that acknowledges language diversity. Is there any in your region/country? If so, what does it state/mandate in regard to linguistic and cultural diversity or access? If language services are mandated, who pays for them? Who monitors the compliance on the part of the organization? What is said (if anything) about quality of service? Is quality measured? If so, how?

Note

1 Throughout the book, we use the results from empirical studies to illustrate the examples. However, because we are discussing stakeholders in abstract and representing many parts of the world, some degree of generalization is unavoidable.

References

Adler, H. (2002). The socio-physiology of caring in the doctor-patient relationship. *Journal of General Internal Medicine*, *17*, 874–881.

American Hospital Association and Institute for Family-Centered Care Resource Guide. (2006). Available at www.ipfcc.org/resources/getting_started.pdf and www.aha.org/toolkitsmethodology/2018-02-08-patient-and-family-centered-care-hospital-self-assessment-inventory (Last accessed January 15, 2018).

Andrulis, D. P., & Brach, C. (2007). Integrating literacy, culture, and language to improve health care quality for diverse populations. *American Journal of Health Behavior*, *31*(1), S122–S133. PMC.

Angelelli, C. V. (2015). *A study on public service translation in cross-border healthcare technical report*. Luxembourg: Publications Office of the European Union. ISBN 978-92-79-47163-6.

———. (2004). *Medical interpreting and cross-cultural communication*. London: Cambridge University Press.

Angelelli, C. V., & Slatyer, H. (2010). Exploring Australian healthcare interpreters perceptions and beliefs on their roles. Paper presented at the *American Translators and Interpreting Studies Bi-Annual Conference*, New York University, New York.

Australian Government. *Department of social services*. Available at www.dss.gov.au/our-responsibilities/settlement-services/programs-policy/settle-in-australia/help-with-english/free-interpreting-service (Last accessed June 2018).

Berwick, D. (2009). What patient-centered should mean: Confessions of an extremist. *Health Affairs*, *28*(4), w555–w565.

Candib, L. (1995). *Medicine and the family: A feminist perspective*. New York: Basic Books.

Chen, A. H. (2004, October 29–November 4). Ask doctor Alice: Is the doctor in? Not if you don't speak English. *Asian Journal Publications*, 23.

Chen, A. H., Youdelman, M. K., & Brooks, J. (2007). The legal framework for language access in healthcare settings: Title VI and Beyond. *Journal of General Internal Medicine*, 22(Suppl 2), 362-367. https://doi.org/10.1007/s11606-007-0366-2

Cohen, G. (2015). *Patients with passports: Medical tourism, law and ethics*. Oxford and New York: Oxford University Press.

Crookes, V., Casey, V., Whitmore, R., Johnston, R., & Snyder, J., et.al. (2015). "They go the extra mile, the extra ten miles. . ." examining Canadian medical tourists' interaction with healthcare workers abroad. In N. Lunt, D. Horsfall, & J. Hanefeld (Eds.), *Handbook on Medical Tourism and Patient Mobility* (Chapter 45, pp. 451–461). Cheltenham, UK and Northampton, MA: Edward Elgar Publishing

Davies, H.T.O., Nutley, S. M., & Mannion, R. (2000). Organisational culture and quality of health care. *BMJ Quality & Safety*, *9*, 111–119.

Department of Health. (2012). EU directive on patients' rights in cross-border healthcare IA no: 6013 [Online]. Available at www.legislation.gov.uk/ukia/2012/42

Entwistle, V. A., Carter, S. M., Cribb, A., & McCaffery, K. (2010). Supporting patient autonomy: The importance of clinician-patient relationships. *Journal of General Internal Medicine*, *25*(7), 741–745. https://doi.org/10.1007/s11606-010-1292-2

Equality Act. (2010). *Equality Act 2010*, c. 15. London: The Stationary Office.

Gee, J. P. (2011). *How to do discourse analysis: A toolkit*. New York and London: Routledge.

Hadler, M. W. (2015). Migration and patient mobility in Latin America. In N. Lunt, D. Horsfall, & J. Hanefeld (Eds.), *Handbook on medical tourism and patient mobility* (pp. 313–323). Cheltenham, UK and Northampton, MA: Edward Elgar Publishing.

Halba, B. (2009). T.I.P.S for intercultural dialogue: T-learning to improve professional skills for intercultural dialogue. Comparative research report. Proposed by FOR.COM (Italy), together with Auxilium (Austria), Iriv (France), HOU (Greece),TEU (Poland), Leonardo da Vinci project (Multilateral project) Institut de Recherche et d'Information sur le Volontariat (IRIV) Paris. Available at www.iriv.net/pdf/Comparative%20research%20report%20-%20Final.pdf (Last accessed May 2018).

Hornberger, J., Gibson, C., Wood, W., Degueldre, C., Corso, I., Palla, B., & Bloch, D. (1996). Eliminating language barriers for non-English-speaking patients. *Medical Care*, *8*, 845–856.

Jacobs, E. A., Lauderdale, D. S., Meltzer, D., Shorey, J. M., Levinson, W., & Thisted, R. A. (2001). Impact of interpreter services on delivery of health care to limited-English-proficiency patients. *Journal of General and Internal Medicine*, *16*, 468–474.

Johnson, B., Abraham, M., Conway, J., Simmons, L., Edgman-Levitan, S., Sodomka, P., Schlucter, J., & Ford, D. (2008). *Partnering with patients and families to design a patient- and family-centered health care system: Recommendations and promising practices*. Bethesda, MD: Institute for Family-Centered Care. Available at www.ipfcc.org/tools/downloads.html

Lee, S. J., Back, A. L., Block, S. D., & Stewart, S. K. (2002). Enhancing physician-patient communication. *Hematology*, *1*, 464–490.

McGraw-Hill Companies. (2002). *McGraw-Hill concise dictionary of modern medicine*. Monterey, CA: McGraw-Hill.

Medical Board of Australia. (2014). *Good medical practice: A code of conduct for doctors in Australia*, p. 5. Available at https://www.medicalboard.gov.au/codes-guidelines-policies/code-of-conduct.aspx

Ministero dell'Interno. (2009). Linee di indirizzo per il riconoscimento della figura professionale del mediatore interculturale. Gruppo di Lavoro Istituzionale per la Promozione della Mediazione Interculturale. Available at www.interno.it/mininterno/export/sites/default/it/assets/files/18/00937_linee_indirizzo_mediatore_interculturale.pdf

Northern Territory Government. (2018). *Interpreting fees*. Available at https://nt.gov.au/community/interpreting-and-translating-services/interpreting-and-translating-service-nt/interpreting-and-translating-fees (Last accessed April 30, 2018).

Official Journal of the European Union. (2011). *Directive 2011/24/EU of the European Parliament and of the Council, of 9 March 2011 on the application of patients' rights in cross-border healthcare* [Online]. Available at http://eur-lex.europa.eu/LexUriServ/LexUriServ.do?uri=OJ:L:2011:088:0045:0065:en:PDF

———. (2010). *The Directive 2010/64/EU of the European Parliament and of the Council of 20 October 2010 on the Right to Interpretation and Translation in Criminal Proceedings*. European Union. Luxembourg: Publications Office of the European Union.

———. (2004). *Regulation (EC) No 883/2004 of the European Parliament and of the Council of 29 April 2004*. Luxembourg: Publications Office of the European Union.

Pruthi, S., Davis, D.M.R., Hucke, D. L., Ripple, F. B., Tatzel, B. S., Dilling, J. A., Santrach, P. J., Bolton, J. W., & Noseworthy, J. H. (2015). Vision, mission, and values: From concept to execution at Mayo Clinic. *Patient Experience Journal*, *2*(2), Article 21, 168–173. Available at: http://pxjournal.org/journal/vol2/iss2/21 (Last accessed April 14, 2018).

Robinson, P., & Tyndale-Biscoe, J. (2012). What makes a top hospital? Organizational culture: Technical report 4. Available at www.chks.co.uk/userfiles/files/CHKS_2012_WMATH_4%20-%20final.pdf. (Last accessed April 14, 2018).

Translation and Interpreting Services. Australian Government. Department of Home Affairs. Available at www.tisnational.gov.au (Last accessed June 2018).

U.S. Code Title 42, Chapter 21, Subchapter § 2000d (1964). Prohibition against exclusion from participation in, denial of benefits of, and discrimination under federally assisted programs on ground of race, color, or national origin.

Wilson, C. (2013). Patient safety and healthcare quality: The case for language access. *International Journal of Health Policy and Management*, *1*(4), 251–253.

Zhou, P., Bundorf, K., Chang, J., Huang, J. X., & Xue, D. (2011). Organizational culture and its relationship with hospital performance in public hospitals in China. *Health Services Research*, *46*(6 Pt 2), 2139–2160. http://doi.org/10.1111/j.1475-6773.2011.01336.x

Further readings/videos

Certification for Medical Interpreters. The national board on www.certifiedmedicalinterpreters.org (Last accessed June 2018).

Crezee, I.H.M. (2013). *Introduction to healthcare for interpreters and translators*. Chapters 7 and 8. Amsterdam and Philadelphia: John Benjamins.

Exworthy, M., & Peckham, S. (2015). Patient's willingness to travel. In N. Lundt, H. Daniel, & H. Johanna (Eds.), *Handbook on medical tourism and patient mobility* (pp. 45–56). Cheltenham, UK and Northampton, MA, USA: Edward Elgar Publishing.

Qualified Interpreters for Quality Health Care: Pt 2 with Subtitles. A joint production of Health Care Interpreter Network and Kaiser Permanente. Available at www.youtube.com/watch?v=lMhlGTLFlb0

3 Understanding interpreter-mediated communication in healthcare

GOALS

In this chapter we will:

- Explore the interaction between patients and providers when working with an interpreter.
- Understand communication in a medical setting: interaction, participants, skills, goals and expectations.

LEARNING OUTCOMES

By successfully completing this chapter, readers will be able to:

- Compare and contrast medical communication in one/two languages and with two/three (or more) co-participants.
- Analyze healthcare interaction and interpreted communicative events.
- Understand medical interpreting as a situated practice.
- Be aware of social factors impacting interpreter-mediated medical communication.
- Describe constraints and opportunities of working in a healthcare setting.
- Understand the possible tension arising from participants' expectations.

This chapter focuses on interpreted medical communication. It presents a more comprehensive approach to healthcare interpreting. This approach calls for a series of focus shifts: from terms to ways of speaking, from a decontextualized assignment to a situated practice and from the interpreter as an isolated player to a member of a team. After reflecting on the profession of healthcare interpreting and the setting in which this situated practice occurs (chapters 1 and 2 respectively), we zoom in to the communicative events in which healthcare interpreters work. We first discuss the interaction between patients and providers sharing a language, the skills needed to communicate and the goals of communication, as well as the participants' expectations of each other and of the encounter and the social factors that impact the interaction. With all of this in mind, we explore how communication occurs across languages and cultures as a healthcare interpreter steps in to facilitate it.

A. Interpreter-mediated communication

A more comprehensive approach to healthcare interpreting

As discussed earlier (Chapter 1), interpreting is a situated practice. As such, interpreting in healthcare should be concerned with the ways of speaking (Hymes 1974), of using language (spoken or sign) and of doing things and interacting of the community in which it is practiced. To do this we reflect on healthcare discourse (whether it materializes as spoken, signed or written text). This means we pay attention to how people interact and talk to each other, when and why they interact and so on. During a medical interview, for example, we pay attention to who says what to whom and why. When we train ourselves to observe interactions, to pay close attention to what people do with language and body while interacting and to listen carefully, we discover a lot more information that helps us with the analysis and the contextualization of the talk.

This analysis, based on ethnography of communication (Hymes 1974), has been used before in interpreting studies to investigate discourse and interpreters' renditions of it. In healthcare communication, for example, the differences between monolingual and interpreted communicative events in healthcare were studied to analyze the role interpreters play in this interaction (Angelelli 2004). In addition, Hymes' s framework was used to study the role of conference interpreters in different discourse communities in which the interpreter is a temporary guest (Angelelli 2000).

Analysis of the healthcare interaction

Analyzing how provider and patient interact, why they interact, who says what to whom and why can be helpful when working in a healthcare setting. This is a way of thinking about healthcare interpreting (as well as interpreting in general) at the macro level. This approach is quite different from the more reductive one that looks at medical interpreting as a decontextualized practice, as a problem, the solution to which is the mastery of terms. Examples of more reductive approaches would be to learn about medical interpreting by studying glossaries or the ethics of the profession, without addressing interpreting skills, the power dynamics in a healthcare setting or the complexity of the role of the healthcare interpreter.

We illustrate this level of detailed analysis using Hymes's concepts of communication and his taxonomy of speaking (Hymes 1974: 5). Hymes, a scholar who revolutionized the way we think about language users in interaction, discusses the following elements in a communicative event. A **speaker** (a user of a language) is quite familiar with the **ways of speaking** that occur in their **speech**

community. This means that, because providers and patients generally belong to two different speech communities (an exception being if a patient is also a healthcare provider or vice versa), each of them is a **fluent speaker** of one of the speech communities and generally not of both. In the healthcare setting we cannot say that both interlocutors (i.e. patient and provider) share a speech community. The speech community of a provider may not be similar to the speech communities of patients seeking care in the healthcare organization. When communication takes place, Hymes distinguishes different layers. Moving from the macro to the micro level, we begin with the speech situation. The **speech situation** is the consultation the medical interview, a conversation between the provider and the patient (both belonging to different speech communities) about, for example, the results of a recent test and the action required on their part. The ***speech event*** is an exchange during that interview, when, for example, the provider explains to the patient the process moving forward. The smallest unit of all is the ***speech act***, which is a remark during that conversation (tone, irony, etc.). For example, the patient uses a specific tone and body language to express sadness and disappointment at the results received or at complexity of the treatment that is advised by the provider.

To contextualize the analysis of a communicative event, according to Hymes's taxonomy of speaking we begin with the setting. The setting means the physical circumstance of an interpreted communicative event, its time and place – for example, a doctor's office in a hospital. The setting, however, does not necessarily mean the same to both interlocutors. While a provider may be familiar with the setting, as it is the place of work the provider navigates daily, a patient may visit for the first time and therefore not know how to get from the doctor's office to the pharmacy, for example.

In terms of analyzing interaction of participants, we pay attention to who is listening and who is speaking, if they take turns equally, if one holds the floor more than the other and so forth. From research on the role of questions in patient/provider interaction (Prince 1986; Angelelli 2004), we learn that providers, not patients, are the ones who ask more questions. This is in line with the power differential between the two participants in the interaction. As to the purpose of the interpreted communicative event, Hymes distinguishes between purposes as outcomes of a speech event as recognized by members of the speech community and purpose as goals, which are the intentions of participants and the strategies they define for the event. If we follow the example of the provider who explains the test to the patient, the provider does so to achieve the outcome of providing information, and his goal in doing so is that the patient makes an informed decision. The patient achieves his goal when he learns the information he needs to understand what needs to be done and his outcome as he makes the decision on how to move forward.

Analysis of the interpreted communicative event

In terms of the message during an interpreted communicative event, we distinguish between form and content (see Chapter 4 for further details). The form of a message is generally obvious to fluent speakers of a community. So, for example, providers are used to using acronyms or speaking in medicalese. So, if a conversation occurs between providers, peers working at the same healthcare organization (HO), there is generally very little need for clarification of the acronyms or the technical terms because they are familiar with them. This is how they speak. The more a way of speaking has become shared and meaningful to a member of a speech community, the less need there is to contextualize it or explain it.

The patient, instead, belongs to a different speech community and, therefore, they generally do not share the ways of speaking of the providers. So when the provider starts explaining the procedure that the patient needs to undergo, the provider may engage in a technical explanation at a level that perhaps is unnecessary or incomprehensible to the patient because of a lack of background knowledge. The same happens with the content of the message that refers to the topic and change of topic. A fluent speaker of a speech community not only understands concepts and terms but also may not require much signposting when a topic is being changed.

Using Hymes's taxonomy, we also pay attention to the tone, manner or spirit of a speech act (e.g. if there is seriousness, sarcasm, humor), the channels through which information is transmitted (oral, written, face-to-face, over the phone, videoconferencing), the forms of the speech (language, dialect, register) and the norms of interaction (the rules governing speaking, i.e. if speakers overlap, as they generally do in Italian or Spanish, or if they take turns, as they generally do in English) and the norms of interpretation (e.g. does one interpret the other's words in the cultural framework of one's own or in the other's?). In addition, participants benefit from recognizing the genre of the communicative event (e.g. if it is a lecture or grand round where the patient's case is presented, or if it is a one-on-one/family discussion on palliative care – as they certainly call for different behaviors on the part of participants in that communicative event). During the encounter, all parties (ideally) are aware of the needs and goals of the others. This applies particularly to the interpreters who, because of their experience and exposure to both cultures (patient's and provider's) and their familiarity with the intricacies of the HO, is able to identify all needs and goals and contribute to achieving them.

Communication between providers and patients

Communication is at the core of the provider-patient relationship. Effective and emphatic communication is necessary to establish trust, which is one of the pillars of provider-patient relationship. Communication is more effective when the parties state things clearly and use simple language (so that comprehension is not hindered), and the provider can meet the patients' needs in an assertive and timely fashion.

Listening to and understanding both the structure of the patient's narrative as well as the content of what a patient is trying to say are important to gain a fuller picture (Nettleton et al. 2005). Patients express themselves in the way they can (some may speak fluently, while others may have some impediments) or they choose to (some may volunteer a lot of information and some may not be willing to talk much). Listening carefully to the way in which patients tell a story about the pain or a symptom they experience, for example, may give the provider important information about both the issue at hand and the way in which the patient organizes their narrative about the issue. So it is as important to capture and reflect on the form in which patients present information as it is to capture and reflect on the content itself (we will discuss this in depth in Chapter 4). Providers are trained in listening and in interpreting what patients are trying to say. This is why it is important that interpreters render to providers the content given by patients without changing its form.

Unlike other types of interpreting (e.g. that which happens in courts of law), medical discourse is not supposed to be adversarial. Rather, it is about achieving mutual understanding in the pursuit of the patient's well-being. For a clinical encounter to be effective, the parties need to communicate verbally very clearly. Even when healthcare providers and patients share the same language, miscommunications happen due to faulty communication and distortions between the two parties (Kaufert and Putsch 1997). Moreover, communication between a physician and a patient becomes even more complicated "when the basic rules that govern communication are uncertain or unclear. This is the case when patients do not speak the same primary language as their physician, or when patients' limited literacy restricts their ability to understand and be understood by their physician."(Roter 2002: 390)

Communicative goals and social factors

As providers and patients communicate, they have several communicative goals they need to achieve. In addition, all parties to communication may have expectations, both of the communicative event and of each other. The patient, for example, may expect the provider to answer questions and have a solution to a problem, while the provider may expect the patient to answer the questions they pose and work toward a solution together (i.e. undergoing treatment).

Additionally, both provider and patient bring their own social factors (socioeconomic status, gender, ethnicity, etc.) to bear in communication. As we have discussed before, patients have their ways of speaking, which may be very different from the HCPs as they belong to different speech communities. For example, when asking a patient to rate or describe his pain, the provider may be exploring issues of intensity and frequency of the reported pain. These may constitute the indicators the provider needs to make decisions on pain management. A colleague belonging to the same speech community as the provider would recognize the purpose of these questions. Instead, when the patient is asked about pain, the patient may tell a story of what he or she can do while in pain, or may narrate how it starts and how it gets dissipated and would certainly not answer in terms of frequency, intensity or duration. The following transcript illustrates some of these different ways of speaking about pain. We enter the conversation when the doctor starts asking information about the pain that brought the patient to the clinic today:

1	D	In a scale from one to ten, how would she rate her pain?
2▶	I	*A ver Señora Rita, en una escala de uno a diez, ¿que número le pondría a su dolor? Por ejemplo, si el uno es que está para irse a bailar y no tiene nada y el diez es que se está muriendo, dónde estaría el dolor?* (Let's see Mrs. Rita, in a scale from one to ten, what number would you assign to your pain? For example, if one is a pain that would allow you to go dancing, you almost don't feel anything and ten is so painful that you are dying from that pain. . .)
3	P	*¿Cómo dice?* (What did you say?)
4	I	*Qué. . . ¿qué número le daría a su dolor?* (What. . . what number would you give to your pain?)
5	P	*Pos. . . a mi me duele mucho.* (Well. . . it hurts a lot.)
6▶	I	*¿Cuánto es mucho señora? ¿Mucho que se está muriendo del dolor?* (How much is a lot Ma'am? Does a lot mean you are dying from the pain?)
7	P	*Pos. . . no. . . muriendo no, pero. . .* (Well. . . no. . . not dying. . . but. . .)
8▶	I	*¿Qué cosas puede hacer con el dolor?* (Which things can you do when you are in pain?)
9	P	*Pos no sé. . . cuando me duele mucho me siento.* (Well, I don't know. . . when it is very hard I sit down.)
10▶	I	*Pero ¿puede cocinar con el dolor?* (But, can you cook when you are in pain?)
11	P	*A veces me pega fuerte y no.* (Sometimes it is very hard and I can't.)
12▶	I	*Y, esas veces, ¿siente como que se va a morir o no tanto?* (And at times, does it feel like you are going to die or it is not so hard?)
13	P	*No, morir no, nomás pega fuerte.* (No, not like I'm going to die, it's just hitting me hard.)
14▶	I	*¿Le ponemos un ocho o un nueve?* (Do we give it an eight or a nine?)
15	P	*Pos yo no sé, pos sí. . .* (I don't know. . . yes.)
16▶	I	When it is most painful it would be close to an eight, doctor.
17	D	Okay.

(Angelelli 2004: 98)

Neither the provider nor the patient specializes in cross-cultural communication and/or they may always be able to discriminate between who is a professional interpreter and who is not. This, as we have discussed in Chapter 1, is a real problem. At times they may have to work with whoever is available to broker communication in order to save time or to get the point across. At times they resort to bilingual employees with limited proficiency in the non-societal language or with no ability to interpret. Or they may resort to family members or friends with limited proficiency in the societal language, for example. In addition, provider and patient may or may not trust family members and, therefore, may or may not prefer family members to perform as interpreters. At times, providers, if in need, may resort to signing and drawing, expecting this can make do for communication.

The provider may be pressed for time, may need an answer to proceed and so forth. The patient may be hoping for rapport, for establishing a relationship and so on. And both parties may have expectations of each other as well as of the interpreter and of whose expectations the interpreter is going to meet first. This is when a professional interpreter can bridge the gaps between each one of their expectations, stating clearly what an interpreter can and cannot do. In addition to goals and expectations, the contextual and personal background of each of the participants impacts communication. The limitations of the current model of healthcare delivery (e.g. pressure for time, long waiting lists), in addition to the social factors of each of the participants (gender, age, race, nationality, socio-economic status, degrees of literacy, etc.) and their communicative needs (establish a diagnosis or prognosis, gain information or advise) also interact with the expectations participants have of each other.

Expectations also impact communication. This has been explained by sociological theories in interpersonal communication. One interesting example is the theory of the significant other (Festinger 1954), which has been discussed in communication and interpersonal relationships frequently as essential in determining how we relate to each other. This theory states that the more central a person may be to the pursuit of one's own goals, the more one is willing to engage, negotiate and spend time and energy with this person because establishing good rapport may be important, unlike a person with whom one may just share an elevator ride (Festinger 1954). In addition, interactions do not happen in a social vacuum. Instead they are affected by the culture of the institution where the communicative event takes places, its rules and regulations. Additionally, healthcare organizations are also part of a larger society. Therefore, the culture, norms and societal blueprints in which healthcare organizations are embedded impact the interaction and communication that takes place in them in them (e.g. communication does not happen in the same way in a private or public hospital in Greece or in Germany).

In this context, participants do their best to accomplish their communicative goals. Providers do their best to achieve goals that line up with their professional mandate (health and well-being of the patient), but they do not specialize in how patients express themselves, how they construct meaning out of the information they receive, their cultures or their beliefs. Some cultural practices that may be acceptable for providers (e.g. discussing organ donation with patient and family members while a terminally ill patient is still alive) may not be acceptable for patients. Patients do their best to comply and participate, but at times they may not be fully aware of the expectations that providers have of them. If, for example, patients come from a culture in which they may do more listening than participating, because they are quiet and do not ask many questions they may be perceived as uninterested in their conditions, when in reality this is not the case. And because many patients recognize it is the provider who has the expertise, they would rather defer to them and not take up the floor so much. Professional interpreters will bridge these gaps of cultural references, ways of speaking and so forth. In the next chapters we will discuss examples of the strategies interpreters have learned to achieve this.

Communicative skills of participants

Communication in a cross-cultural setting is more successful when the healthcare provider is able to use their communication skills during the encounter, especially in the phases of patient assessment and elicitation of information in order to understand the patient's perspective of symptoms and explanatory health belief. When the provider has these skills, usually the result is increased patient satisfaction, trust and compliance (Ferguson and Candib 2002). Providers must be aware that patients of different ethnic backgrounds differ in the way they want to be told about their medical condition, especially if it involves some bad news. Some cultures believe that the mere fact of stating or discussing bad news is in itself a precursor of something bad. Most patients prefer to be told bad news, to receive all available information and options about their disease and treatment options (Lee et al. 2002). Therefore, these patients would expect the physicians to know about, and openly address, cross-cultural differences in patients' preferences about the delivery of bad news. However, not all patients may be explicit about these preferences. Even patients who are interested in specific information, such as prognosis, may not ask questions. Therefore, providers should not assume that patients automatically would state aloud their questions when asked "Do you have any questions for me?" or "Would you like to ask any questions at this point?" And, most importantly, providers should not conclude that patients are not interested in their health if they do not ask questions. This simply shows a cultural difference and not a lack of interest in providing answers and helping providers. This is another example of parties who do not share a speech community or expectations of each other.

Impact of language barriers and cultural gaps

While findings from most studies in healthcare communication support the idea that professional interpreters are more likely to bridge the gaps in healthcare access for patients who do not speak the societal language, they have also demonstrated the persistence of poor communication skills on the part of the physicians, in spite of the presence of interpreters. Poorly organized medical-language services can discourage linguistically diverse patients from seeking appropriate healthcare. Undoubtedly, both patients and providers benefit from professional interpreter services while trying to communicate. However, it is also true that the patients are the most vulnerable parties in the equation and, therefore, patients are the ones who assume most of the negative consequences (avoidable morbidity or mortality) related to poor outcomes resulting from ineffective communication when interpreter services are not used or are used improperly (see, e.g., Ferguson and Candib 2002).

Patients have limited ability in the societal language and because of their language or their inability to use the societal language (generally referred to as language barriers),[1] they cannot benefit from the fundamental interaction between HCP and patients (Jacobs et al. 2001). Because language and communication are at the core of healthcare delivery, language problems can hinder multiple aspects of it, from access to health status, use of health services and health outcomes. It has been reported that patients who are not proficient in the societal language "are less likely to engender empathic responses from physicians, less likely to establish rapport with physicians, less likely to receive sufficient information, and less likely to be encouraged to participate in medical decision making" (Ferguson and Candib 2002: 353). In addition, patients' inability to speak the same language as their physicians or other providers compromises their access to care and the quality of that care (Hornberger et al. 1996).

Linguistically diverse patients who cannot access the societal language have fewer primary care visits and receive fewer preventive services, which leads to a poorer health status. It is not clear who is responsible for this: the patient or the provider. On the other hand, patients in cross-linguistic encounters are more likely to make emergency room visits. Some authors would explain this by saying that the patients' inability to access the societal language causes them to delay the visit to healthcare providers as much as they can until a problem becomes severe (Rivadeneyra et al. 2000). They prefer to wait instead of having to try to describe their symptoms to someone who speaks a different language. The communication barrier between non-English-speaking patients and their healthcare providers extends beyond just language difficulties. It is also a problem of trust, inviting both physician and patient to change their behavior in subtle ways in order to develop a trusting relationship. Not having a trusting relationship because of different languages (which can be bridged with interpreting) increases the likelihood of the physician misunderstanding the patient's description of her symptoms and decreases the probability that the patient will adhere to the physician's recommendations.

Ideally, all patients would be cared for by physicians who speak their language and share their culture (Flores 2000; Rivadeneyra et al. 2000). Being able to communicate directly improves patient compliance and understanding of their disease (Manson 1988). According to Ferguson and Candib (2002), "the literature calls for a more diverse physician workforce since minority patients are more likely to choose minority physicians, to be more satisfied by language-concordant relationships, and to feel more connected and involved in decision making with racially-concordant physicians" (p. 353). Because this is not always possible, communication problems between doctors and patients who speak different languages are seen nationwide (Marcus 2003). The quality of the physician-patient relationship affects the diagnosis, treatment and recovery of patients. Some authors point out that the clinical outcome of patients who do not speak the societal language is improved by good communication (Kuo and Fagan 1999; Rivadeneyra et al. 2000).

When they are able to communicate with their healthcare providers, patients develop a better understanding of their disease and they comply more with the proposed treatment. Doctors, patients and their family members are able to work together successfully thanks to a good communication. To achieve this, various strategies for improving access for patients who do not speak the societal language have been formulated: (1) care by physicians or medical residents who are bilingual; (2) use of bilingual support staff; (3) use of bilingual employees who interpret in addition to their regular work; (4) use of professional interpreters; and (5) use of the speakerphone to provide remote language interpreting (Barnett 2002; Ferguson and Candib 2002; García 2000; Kuo and Fagan 1999). The use of these strategies is especially important during the medical interview, which is discussed in the next section.

The medical interview

Most of the interactions between physicians and patients are in the form of an interview. The patient interview is "the primary way of obtaining comprehensive information about the patient in order to provide effective patient-centered care" (Srivastava 2014). It allows the healthcare provider to obtain information from the patient about the specific complaint but also the medication taken, the allergies, adverse reactions, the family (medical) history and the social environment of the patient. To achieve this goal, it is necessary that healthcare providers and healthcare interpreters have good communication skills. The following features have been identified in medical interviews: (1) the skills used by a clinician (e.g. sustained listening, closed questions, gentle commands or invitations to talk); (2) the functions of the interview (e.g. data retrieval, building rapport with the patient, seeking to know the patient's values); and (3) the data desired (patient's personal story, the chief complaint [cardinal symptom], symptom descriptors, etc.) (Platt 2014).

In addition to the skills, functions and data discussed above, different phases of the interview have also been identified. These phases constitute the typical structure of a medical interview. In their study of verbal behaviors in over 2,000 medical consultations, Byrne and Long (1976) identified six phases: (1) relating to the patient, (2) discovering the reason for attendance, (3) conducting a verbal or physical examination or both, (4) consideration of the patient's condition, (5) detailing treatment or further investigation, and (6) terminating. Taking a closer look at each phase, we see their parts. Research on medical communication allows us to identify the parts (and goals) of the phases of medical interviews. Let's take a look at the opening phase (Binder 2010: 12):

1. Creating a working relationship with the family and the patient, one based on mutual respect and trust.
2. Establishing emotional safety.
3. Checking own internal emotional experience.
4. Activating the family to give their perception of the problem.
5. Evaluating the *process* of the interview itself.
6. Obtaining the family's full agenda, organizing and prioritizing it, and explaining your plan for the rest of the interview to the family.

In each of the parts, and during the interview as a whole, participants (the provider and the patient in a monolingual interview, or the provider, the patient and the interpreter in an interpreted one) have goals that they need to accomplish.

Interpreter-mediated communication for providers and patients

Specifically, when discussing provider-patient communication mediated by an interpreter, it is important to distinguish two terms: interaction and relationship. Given that effective communication between patient and provider is key to developing a therapeutic relationship, the healthcare interpreter needs to pay special attention to how the interpreted interaction is managed so that it contributes to the development of the provider-patient relationship.

Role of communication

Provider-patient relationships are dependent on effective communication. In the case of linguistically diverse patients, this means that these patients need to have access to the different strategies described earlier in order to communicate adequately with their healthcare providers (Jacobs et al. 2001). The health status of these patients could be compromised if the communication process is put at risk. Even when everything is fine and the parties understand each other well, cross-language encounters are by nature slower and less precise than same-language medical encounters. Physicians are aware that a relationship-centered approach is linked to better medical outcomes. However, some physicians cite lack of time as a problem in using such an approach with their patients, especially if they do not speak the societal language (Rivadeneyra et al. 2000). This raises the question, given the complexity and numerous constraints of a medical encounter, can a patient-centered relationship ever develop between a provider and a patient who do not share language or culture? A relationship is quite different from an interaction or an encounter. What can be done to bridge this gap that exists in communication between providers and patients? In order to determine a diagnosis and develop a therapeutic plan, the physicians rely on information gathered during the medical history. Information gathering is more challenging when the physician and patient do not have a common language. This is one of the reasons why a professional medical interpreter is needed for precise and effective information gathering, which can only be helpful in building relationship across languages. Trust can be built and misunderstandings can be avoided with effective communication.

Both providers and interpreters need to understand the importance of being patient-centered or perhaps, even more important, of being person-focused. Indeed,

> both patient-centered and person-focused care are important, but they are different. In contrast to patient-centered care (at least as described in the current literature with assessments that are visit-based), person-focused care is based on accumulated knowledge of people, which provides the basis for better recognition of health problems and needs over time and facilitates

> appropriate care for these needs in the context of other needs. That is, it specifically focuses on the whole person.
>
> (Starfield 2011: 63)

Such focus improves the quality of the care as it considers the person as a whole and over time.

If the building of a relationship depends on communication, and if the essence of a relationship is described by the association between two entities, in an interpreted medical encounter, then, we should ask ourselves the following questions. How can a relationship be established between provider and patient/person when there is a third party involved? How is the presence of a family member or interpreter affecting the establishment of such relationship? When an interpreter is involved, who is the relationship between? Doctor and interpreter? Doctor and patient? Patient and interpreter? Or doctor, patient and interpreter? Can a three-party interaction, a communicative *pas de trois* (Wadensjö 1998), be as efficient for a relationship-centered medical visit as a two-party interaction? And would the possibility of the relationship even exist without the interpreter? And in a three-party relationship, can the formation of alliances between any two members of the three-party interaction be avoided? Sometimes? Always? Maybe they do not need to be avoided? It all depends on the goal of the alliance.

Blanket statements may not be helpful. If the relationship is to safeguard the well-being of the patient, the three parties need to be part of the alliance, as in the *pas de trois*. However, what if the relationship is about bonding over a favorite dish from the country of origin that the interpreter and the patient share, and if this bonding helps build trust, and does not interfere with the patient/provider communication? In the case of hospitals having interpreter services, it is not uncommon to hear that when satisfied with the interpreting during an encounter, a provider sometimes requests the same interpreter for the next cross-linguistic medical interaction. The same holds true for the patient. Sometimes patients request interpreters with whom they can communicate more effectively.

As we have seen, communicating through an interpreter can be a double-edged sword. When used improperly, it becomes a hindrance to establishing a therapeutic patient-provider relationship. On the other hand, effective communication brokered through an interpreter can have a profoundly positive impact on the patient and their well-being. As it maximizes the exchange of information between provider and patient, it may increase trust, relationship building and, as a result, compliance.

Social factors, communication and relationships

Disparities in health outcomes among ethnic minority and racial groups have become increasingly clear. Research has shown how differences in race, ethnicity and language appear to affect the provider-patient relationship (Ferguson and Candib 2002). These authors, among others, believe that the doctor-patient relationship may be important in explaining such disparities even though the reasons for such disparities remain unclear. According to Flores (2000):

> failure to consider a patient's cultural and linguistic issues can result in inaccurate histories, decreased satisfaction with care, non-adherence, poor continuity of care, less preventive screening, miscommunication, difficulties with informed consent, inadequate analgesia, a lower likelihood of having a primary care provider, decreased access to care, use of harmful remedies, delayed immunizations, and fewer prescriptions.
>
> (p. 21)

Linguistic minority patients are less likely to engender an empathic response from physicians. They have difficulties in establishing rapport with physicians, which translates into insufficient information being exchanged between them. As a result, the patient is less encouraged to participate in medical decision-making, and the clinicians sometimes provide a lower quality of care to patients from different cultures (Ferguson and Candib 2002; Flores 2000). In addition, patients who cannot speak the societal language well receive less than optimal healthcare and are at greater risk of not receiving preventive care and other services. They are likely to find their providers less friendly and less respectful (Jacobs et al. 2001). As a result, linguistic minority patients have less desire to seek out the same provider and, consequently, to establish trusting, professional relationships (Rivadeneyra et al. 2000).

In sum, it is important to bear in mind that professional relationships based on shared work experiences may develop among the interpreter and the other staff members. In addition, as discussed above, in the case of a hospital that provides language services, it is not unusual for patients to request a specific staff interpreter once they have worked together several times. The same holds true for providers. Patients may want to work with the same provider they trust, as this means continuity and consistency in their care. Providers may want to work with the same interpreter for the same reasons.

Other factors influencing HCP/HI/patient relationship

In addition to the use of different languages and the ability to communicate more or less efficiently, there are other factors that impact the quality and delivery of healthcare. A patient's health beliefs and practices are the product of a combination of normative cultural values together with personal experience and perceptions (Flores 2000; Hornberger et al. 1996). In other words, provider and patient may share the same language but may have important differences in their cultural norms. These can lead to miscommunication and misunderstanding. The majority of physicians need to be more effective in developing relationships in their communication with ethnic and racial minority patients (Ferguson and Candib 2002: 353). Providers must be aware of and respond appropriately to a patient's normative cultural values. Otherwise, they may cause a variety of adverse clinical consequences which may have a negative impact on a patient's access, health status, use of health services and health outcomes (Flores 2000). Roter (2002) reminds us that "complex challenges are presented to physicians when assumptions regarding the social rules that govern communication are uncertain or unclear, as in the case of cross-cultural communication" (p. 390).

Influence of culture on overall quality of healthcare

Culture can have major clinical consequences in the patient-physician relationship (Flores 2000). Even without language differences, effective communication may be hindered by cultural differences, which leads to misunderstandings. The same information can be understood differently depending on how it is presented (Lee et al. 2002). People are defined by their language, among other factors. Language is what makes them members of a language group. They are also defined by a framework of beliefs, symbols and values often expressed through distinct language or the unique use of a common language: that is culture. Additionally, language-linked cultural norms may apply to broad categories of patients, including those identified by their gender, ethnicity, sexual orientation, age cohort or religious beliefs (Roter 2002). Physicians often find themselves in situations in which their cultural beliefs and values differ from their patients', and vice versa, which may hinder the establishment of the cooperative partnership (Lee et al. 2002).

In addition to culture, there is the ability to differentiate between a competent and an incompetent language service provider. Even when interpreters may be available, there is often little or no standardization in interpreter education/training, assessment of competence, or training for healthcare providers on how to work with an interpreter (Baker et al. 1998). In the United States, for example, several states have passed laws or established regulations requiring providers to have interpreters or bilingual staff available for patients who need them (MMIA 1995; California Healthcare Interpreter Association [CHIA] 2002). "These laws and regulations, however, do not define what constitutes adequate screening, testing, training, and proficiency for interpreters," assert Baker et al. (1998: 1469). Select policy-making bodies have attempted to define the standards of practice and role of the interpreter in the medical setting. The goal is to help decrease interpreting errors and to diminish behaviors that adversely affect the patient-provider relationship. Similarly, in the UK, the National Register of Public Service Interpreters maintains a public register of professionally qualified interpreters. Every interpreter in the registry has met the standards set for education, training and practice in the public service, but screening/testing has not been studied.

Impact of healthcare interpreting

When an interpreter is assigned to a medical encounter, both practical and ethical problems may arise (Kaufert and Putsch 1997). The presence or absence of an interpreter impacts the encounter in various ways. The presence of an interpreter reduces the direct verbal communication and nonverbal reciprocity between doctor and patient, thus rendering the encounter less personal and decreasing the patient's sense of connection to their provider. This is especially the case when providers have not been taught how to use an interpreter (Baker et al. 1998; Rivadeneyra et al. 2000). Findings from a study conducted by Baker et al. (1998) established that the presence of a third party may negatively affect the relationship (because of a decreased sense of privacy and intimacy between patient and physician), even when the interpreter and the clinician may have optimal training in how to work in this situation. The authors found that patients who communicated through an interpreter were less likely to know their diagnosis and more likely to say they wished the provider had explained better, whereas patients who were able to communicate directly with their provider demonstrated more satisfaction. Patients who communicated through an interpreter also rated their provider as less friendly, less respectful, less concerned with the patient as a person and less likely to take measures to make the patient feel comfortable.

On the other hand, according to Jacobs et al. (2001), interpreting services have the potential to increase provision of clinical, therapeutic and preventive services through three mechanisms: (1) enhanced patient and physician understanding; (2) enhanced physician-patient trust; and (3) patient satisfaction. Enhanced patient and physician understanding motivates patients to make and keep appointments. It also gives physicians more confidence in their diagnoses and in the patient's understanding of the risks and benefits of a particular treatment. Patients are more likely to get their prescriptions filled because they understand both the purpose of the treatment and the instructions for taking the medication. Enhanced physician-patient trust is established by effective communication. This two-way trust is dependent upon understanding, caring, clear communication, partnership building and question answering.

Therefore, even when difficulties may arise when communication is facilitated by an interpreter, even greater negative consequences can be seen when an interpreter is needed but not called or available. Research conducted in a large staff model health-maintenance organization shows that professional interpreter services increase delivery of healthcare to patients who cannot access the societal language. Patients who use the interpreter services in this healthcare organization have a significantly greater increase in office visits, prescription writing and prescription filling compared to a control group (Jacobs et al. 2001).

Therefore, as stated earlier, linguistic differences are not a barrier or a problem per se. They become a problem when they are not dealt with appropriately and professionally. Linguistic differences are a fact of life. Many institutions around the world deal with language differences by relying extensively on untrained interpreters (Ginsberg et al. 1995 in Baker 1998). The National Public Health and Hospital Institute in the United States conducted a survey in 83 public and private hospitals; the survey results showed that less than one-fourth of hospitals offer any interpreting training for their staff. Only nine hospitals trained their volunteer interpreters; the other 74 use people untrained in interpreting, the so called ad hoc interpreters: patients, family, friends and hospital staff. As many authors argue, this practice often results in errors in interpreting (omissions, additions and substitutions) and condensations of what was said by both the clinician and the patient (Flores 2000; Baker et al. 1998; Jacobs et al. 2001).

Baker et al. 1998 conducted a study on behaviors of family members acting as interpreters. It was found that family members acting as interpreters volunteered their own information and opinion. Frequently they responded directly to questions without allowing the patient to answer. In addition, they failed to interpret certain patient comments and questions. Inadequate interpreting also impaired patient-provider communication about diagnosis and treatment, as some physician's questions were misinterpreted or not interpreted at all. Ad hoc interpreters occasionally make behavioral mistakes that may affect both patient and physician satisfaction. Additionally, ad hoc interpreters sometimes are family members who accompany patients, especially elderly patients, to their medical visits. Some researchers (Campbell et al. 2002) argue that patients accompanied by a family member acting as interpreter behave differently than unaccompanied patients. Differences in reactions and behaviors were observed in relation to their medical problems, family relationships, functional abilities and attitudes toward family involvement in their care. The mere presence of a third party, of someone other than the physician and patient, during the visits introduces a new set of psychosocial factors into the equation, posing a risk for the physician-patient relationship.

An important part of establishing a relationship in many cultures is eye contact. In an interpreter-mediated encounter, often both HCPs and patients look at the person doing the interpreting during the clinical encounter instead of looking at one another. The lack of eye contact not only may put distance between them but it also may lessen providers' awareness of nonverbal clues about patients' thoughts and feelings. This could have adverse consequences on the taking of the clinical history. Ad hoc services have many negative clinical consequences including "reduced trust in physicians, lower patient satisfaction, and breach of patient confidentiality, inaccurate communication, misdiagnosis, inadequate or inaccurate treatment, and reduced quality of care" (Jacobs et al. 2001: 469). On the other hand, a study by Kuo and Fagan (1999) showed that some patients prefer when family members or friends interpret for them instead of unfamiliar interpreters; they derive a great deal of comfort when they can express what they feel to someone who is not just from their culture, but is someone they know. Ad hoc interpreters may bring other advantages: they are inexpensive and readily available.

Another benefit of having family members who accompany the patient act as interpreters is that they can also assist the patient with tasks such as arranging transportation and follow-up visits; they play roles that go beyond providing language assistance. From the outset of the medical encounter, the healthcare interpreters introduce themselves and explain their role. Family members may not do that because they do not follow interpreters' protocol. Instead, healthcare interpreters manage the content, the form and the flow of information during the encounter, closure activities and patient referral to auxiliary services (Baker et al. 1998). They also manage the dynamics of the medical encounter by encouraging patient and doctor to address each other directly. It is important to understand that building trust is just a part of the job of the healthcare interpreter.

Cultural differences as well as language proficiency may independently influence patients' expectations for satisfactory medical care. Jacobs et al. remind us to be mindful of the fact that the findings of a few studies may not be generalizable to all clinics or all languages. However, the findings of these studies cannot be ignored. The fact remains that cultural, educational and economic barriers exist for many linguistically diverse patients. As the authors state, "providing these patients with the means to inform [their healthcare providers] about their symptoms and concerns and to navigate health care delivery systems is an important step toward improving their health" (2001: 473).

B. Research, observe and reflect

Go to your local clinic/hospital. Alternatively look for samples of medical interviews on the internet (we suggest a few YouTube interviews in the Further Readings section). Identify the various components of the patient interview. Compare the various approaches you see and reflect about which one you feel is most effective. Do you feel the interview you have observed meets the needs of the healthcare provider? Of the patient? What probing question do you think was particularly effective?

C. Journal writing

In this chapter we have discussed communication between patient and provider facilitated by an interpreter. We have learned about looking at interpreting as a communicative event and as a situated practice. We have studied how different social factors affect communication (both monolingual and bilingual). In this journal entry, we would like you to reflect on all of this and what it means for you, as the healthcare interpreter, in the moment of facilitating communication. Think of what it means to work across different discourse communities, different levels of education, socio-economic status, race, ethnicity, age and gender. How do all of these factors play out in communication? In what ways can we achieve understanding on healthcare issues among people whose conceptualization of health and well-being could be different? Think if your views on healthcare interpreting have remained unchanged or not after reading this chapter. Discuss your reasons in this entry.

D. Further tasks

1 Communicative goals and social factors: Go back to the transcript about the pain scale. Imagine you are the interpreter in that encounter. Reread it and point at what parts of the transcript can tell you important things about the two parties. Can you think of other ways of working with this question? Think about other cultures/languages you know. How do they conceptualize,

discuss and deal with pain? Compare and contrast patients and providers from at least two different parts of the world.

2 Go to Chapter 6. Look at the transcript in which Marta is interpreting (section B). Point at the turns that can give you information about communicative goals and social factors.

Note

1 Many languages are spoken in our diverse societies today. Languages are different. This does not mean languages are a barrier or a problem per se. A barrier can be lifted and a problem can be solved. By taking action, we change current power and access inequalities among linguistic groups/peoples. As result of inequalities, some linguistic groups gain access to healthcare services and others do not. By labeling diversity or differences as a problem or a barrier, societies find a justification to avoid the expense of paying professionals (interpreters, translators or mediators, according to the communicative needs). Professional services exist, and they bridge language differences. The problem is what we as societies choose to do or not to do about language differences.

References

Angelelli, C. (2004). *Medical interpreting and cross-cultural communications*. Cambridge: Cambridge University Press.

———. (2000). Interpreting as a communicative event: A look through Hymes' lenses. *Meta: Journal des Traducteurs*, *45*, 580–592.

Barnett, S. (2002). Cross-cultural communication with patients who use American sign language. *Family Medicine*, *34*(5), 376–382.

Binder, J. (2010). *Pediatric interviewing: A practical, relationship-based approach*. New York, Dordrecht, Heidelberg and London: Humana Press c/o Springer. doi:10.1007/978-1-60761-256-8_2

Byrne, P. S., & Long, B.E.I. (1976). *Doctors talking to patients: A study of the verbal behaviours of doctors in consultation*. London: Department of Health and Social Security.

Campbell, T. L., McDaniel, S. H., Cole-Kelly, K., Hepworth, J., & Lorenz, A. (2002). Family interviewing: A review of the literature in primary care. *Family Medicine*, *34*(5), 312–318.

CHIA (California Healthcare Interpreters Association). (2002). *California standards for healthcare interpreters: Ethical principles, protocols, and guidance on roles and intervention*. Sacramento: California Endowment.

Ferguson, W. J., & Candib, L. M. (2002). Culture, language, and the doctor-patient relationship. *Family Medicine*, *34*(5), 353–361.

Festinger, L. (1954). A theory of social comparison processes. *Human Relations*, *7*, 117–140.

Flores, G. (2000). Culture and the patient-physician relationship: Achieving cultural competency in health care. *Journal of Pediatrics*, *136*, 14–23.

García, A. (2000). Remote telephone interpreting system implemented at Santa Clara Valley Medical. *CHIA Newsletter*, *2*(2), 1.

Ginsberg, C., Martin, V. A., Andrulis, D., Shaw-Taylor, Y., & McGregor, C. (1995). *Interpretation and translation services in health care: A survey of US public and private teaching hospitals*. Washington, DC: National Public Health and Hospital Institute.

Hornberger, J., Gibson, C., Wood, W., Degueldre, C., Corso, I., Palla, B., & Bloch, D. (1996). Eliminating language barriers for non-English-speaking patients. *Medical Care*, *8*, 845–856.

Hymes, D. (1974). *Foundations in sociolinguistics*. Philadelphia, NJ: University of Pennsylvania Press, Inc.

Jacobs, E. A., Lauderdale, D. S., Meltzer, D., Shorey, J. M., Levinson, W., & Thisted, R. A. (2001). Impact of interpreter services on delivery of health care to Limited-English-proficiency patients. *Journal of General and Internal Medicine*, *16*, 468–474.

Kaufert, J., & Putsch, R. (1997). Communication through interpreters in healthcare: ethical dilemmas arising from differences in class, culture, language and power. *The Journal of Clinical Ethics*, *8*(1), 71–87.

Kuo, D., & Fagan, M. (1999). Satisfaction with methods of Spanish interpretation in an ambulatory care clinic. *Journal of General Internal Medicine*, *14*, 547–550.

Lee, S. J., Back, A. L., Block, S. D., & Stewart, S. K. (2002). Enhancing physician-patient communication. *Hematology*, *1*, 464–490.

Manson, A. (1988). Language concordance as a determinant of patient compliance and emergency room use in patients with asthma. *Medical Care*, *26*, 1119–1128.

Marcus, E. (2003). When a patient is lost in the translation. *New York Times*, New York: F7.

Massachusetts Medical Interpreters Association MMIA. (1995). *Medical interpreting standards of practice*. Boston: Massachusetts Medical Interpreters Association.

Nettleton, S., Watt, I., O'Malley, L., & Duffey, P. (2005, February). Understanding the narratives of people who live with medically unexplained illness. *Patient Education Counselling*, *56*(2), 205–210.

Platt, F. (2014). *Field guide to the difficult patient interview*, 2nd edition. Baltimore, MD: Lippincott Williams and Willkens.

Prince, C. (1986). *Hablando con el doctor: Communication problems between doctors and their Spanish-speaking patients*. Ph.D. diss., Stanford University, Stanford, CA.

Rivadeneyra, R., Elderkin-Thompson, V., Silver, R. C., & Waitzkin, H. (2000). Patient centeredness in medical communication literature. *Archives of Family Medicine*, *6*, 279–283.

Roter, D. (2002). Three blind men and an elephant: Reflections on meeting the challenges of patient diversity in primary care practice. *Family Medicine*, *34*(5), 390–393.

Srivastava, S. B. (2014). The patient interview. In C. D. Lauster & S. B. Srivastava (Eds.), *Fundamental skills for patient care in pharmacy practice*. Burlington: Jones and Bartlett Learning. Available at http://samples.jbpub.com/9781449652722/9781449645106_ch01_001_036.pdf (Last accessed May 14, 2018).

Starfield, B. (2011). Is patient-centered care the same as person-focused care? In J. Perm, *The Permanente Journal*, *15*(2, Spring), 63–69. Available at www.ncbi.nlm.nih.gov/pmc/articles/PMC3140752/ Copyright © 2011 (Last accessed June 4, 2018).

Wadensjö, C. (1998). *Interpreting as interaction*. New York: Addison Wesley Longman Inc.

Further readings and resources

Amato, A. (2007). The interpreter in multi-party medical encounters. In C. Wadensjö, B. E. Dimitrova, & A.-L. Nilsson (Eds.), *The critical link 4: Professionalization of interpreting in the community* (pp. 27–38). John Benjamins Publishing Company.

Baker, M. (2006). Contextualization in translator- and interpreter-mediated events. In M. Baker, *Translation and Context*, *38*(3), 321–337.

Baraldi, C., & Gavioli, L. (2014). Are close renditions the golden standard? Some thoughts on translating accurately in healthcare interpreter-mediated interaction, *The Interpreter and Translator Trainer*, *8*(3), 336–353.

Cirillo, L. (2010). Managing affect in interpreter-mediated institutional talk: Examples from the medical setting. In Jan Cambridge, *Interpreting in the Public Services*, (14), 55–79.

Gavioli, L. (2012). Minimal responses in interpreter-mediated medical talk. In C. Baraldi & L. Gavioli (Eds.), *Coordinating participation in dialogue interpreting* (pp. 201–228). John Benjamins Publishing Company.

Meyer, B., Apfelbaum, B., Pöchhacker, F., & Bischoff, A. (2001). Analysing interpreted doctor-patient communication from the perspectives of linguistics, interpreting studies and health sciences. In L. Brunette, G. L. Bastin, I. Hemlin, H. Clarke (Eds.), *The critical link 3: Interpreters in the community* (pp. 67–79). John Benjamins Publishing Company.

Meyer, B., Pawlack, B., & Kliche, O. (2010). Family interpreters in hospitals: Good reasons for bad practice? In: R. Antonini, *Child Language Brokering: Trends and Patterns in Current Research*, (10), 297–324.

Niemants, N.S.A. (2013). From role-playing to role-taking: Interpreter's role(s) in healthcare. In C. Schäffner, K. Kredens, & Y. Fowler (Eds.), *Interpreting in a changing landscape: Selected papers from critical link 6* (pp. 305–319). John Benjamins.

Tipton, R. (2010). On trust: Relationships of trust in interpreter-mediated social work encounters. In M. Baker, M. Calzada Pérez, & M. Olohan (Eds.), *Text and context: Essays on translation and interpreting in honour of Ian Mason*. Manchester UK and Kinderhook, NY: St. Jerome Publishing.

Zimányi, K. (2013)."Somebody has to be in charge of a session": On the control of communication in interpreter-mediated mental health encounters. *Translation and Interpreting Studies*, *8*(1), 94–111.

Other resources

Patient Interview Complete Interview Harvard University OSCE Guide. This video describes the various phases of an interview.

www.youtube.com/watch?v=L70uIpykvow

Nurse-patient interview. This video shows poor skills on the part of the nurse. www.youtube.com/watch?v=oHreolyshYY

Medical specialties and ways of speaking

Specialty profiles: This series of short interviews asks specialists what their practice is like.

Read more profiles in *AMA Wire*'s "Shadow Me" Specialty Series to learn additional insights from physicians in such specialties as infectious disease medicine, adolescent medicine, physical medicine and rehabilitation, radiology and orthopedic surgery, among others.

In each of these interviews, physicians are asked a series of questions such as "Give three adjectives to describe the qualities that a specialist in the field should exhibit," "What good readings should a student in this specialty not miss" and so forth.

https://wire.ama-assn.org/search/site/Shadow%20me

https://wire.ama-assn.org/delivering-care/cardiovascular-health

4 Understanding content and form in interpreter-mediated medical communication

GOALS

In this chapter we will:

- Become aware of the differences between message content and form.
- Learn about interpreting in mental health.
- Explore the impact of technology on healthcare interpreters.

LEARNING OUTCOMES

By successfully completing this chapter, we will be able to:

- Prepare for an assignment.
- Learn to distinguish between implicit and explicit content.
- Identify when to seek clarification.
- Analyze the influence of the form of a message and the options for the interpreter.
- Learn to deal with content and form using different technologies.

In this chapter we focus on interpreted communicative events. Our goal is to study the content of a medical consultation and the form in which the content is discussed – in other words, the "what" and the "how" of these events. We do this by reviewing the existing literature on the topic and exploring empirical data from authentic bilingual-healthcare consultations mediated by interpreters in healthcare settings. One of the biggest challenges in healthcare provision, especially when more than one language is involved, is the provision of mental health care. We briefly review the research on interpreters working with patients diagnosed with mental health conditions to reflect the peculiarities of interpreting in this specialty. We also look at how different technologies impact interpreter-mediated communication.

A. Meaning and understanding: do the same things mean the same to all?

When studying a doctor and a patient interacting, it becomes evident that, in this private encounter, the interpreter multitasking occurs at different levels. Patients, providers and interpreters vary in how they conceptualize the provider-patient relationship and the main goal of an interview (the limited time they have together). They may have different expectations of the encounter. Expectations may vary from establishing rapport or creating trust to facilitating mutual understanding of a plan of action, transferring technical knowledge or providing access to information. Patients and providers also vary in how they talk about and react to issues such as death, cognitive impairment or pain. For example, a patient scared about death may not even be able to talk about it; the provider, being pragmatic, may see the need to discuss palliative care. Or, a patient may feel devastated or lost when diagnosed with Alzheimer's disease; the provider may emphasize the importance of being ready for what is coming by making the necessary arrangements. And as the provider tests the pain intensity or frequency, for example, the patient may be screaming with pain or simply being stoic and pretending pain does not hurt, when in reality it does; the provider may read the reactions of the former as dramatic and the latter as not being interested in their own well-being.

The truth is that interpreters juggle a complex situated practice in all its entirety. They not only deal with the two languages and cultures and the information processing of content and form in real time, but they also deal with human interaction in one of the most private and precious matters of humans: their own lives and well-being. Although the practice of HI needs to be segmented into its components (skills and competencies in interpreting, knowledge of medical issues and settings, ethics, interpersonal skills, etc.) to make learning and teaching of interpreting feasible, the importance of all the components and the ability to juggle all of them simultaneously and in real time should always be acknowledged (in Chapters 5 and 6, we discuss specific skills in detail). This acknowledgment is key when dealing with stressful situations or stressed clients. In this chapter, we look at the general skills of understanding and communicating messages, as they are the basis of interpreting.

Interpreters work for both patients and providers. As we discussed in the previous chapter, patients and providers belong to different discourse communities, and so does the interpreter. Through their education, healthcare providers have been socialized into a medical discourse community (see Chapter 3) and have learned to speak in a specific way about illness, health, life or death (even when they do so only in their culture and their language). They have also acquired ways of conceptualizing and discussing life and death. Interpreters, on the other hand, have not been socialized into the same speech community (as also discussed in Chapter 3). Their ways of conceptualizing or discussing life or death, for example, may be different. Although interpreters can certainly interpret the content and form of a message about life or death, they may or may not be affected by the message content in the same way as the healthcare provider. Although interpreters may have worked in a hospital, may have visited it or may even have been patients themselves, in general, interpreters speak about their own health matters in different ways than providers do. Healthcare interpreters, therefore, in addition to working across languages and cultures navigate two different speech communities as they go about doing their work in a medical setting.

Interpreters are aware of the differences arising from how the two main interlocutors for whom they work, talk/sign behave. When interpreters have not had the chance to study and reflect on interpersonal communication or discourse and interaction, they build knowledge out of their own experience. Many times, because of how busy they are, interpreters do not have a chance to reflect on their experiences and on the relevancy of what they are learning from the experiences. Experiential knowledge is valuable and should not be dismissed, but it needs to be acknowledged as such, to avoid generalizing what is not generalizable. During an interview with an interpreter (a physician in his own country) working as a staff interpreter in a hospital, he reflects on the difference in how physicians and interpreters react to difficult situations and speak about his experience wearing both hats:

> *Hay situaciones en donde el médico por razones de exceso de trabajo, por situaciones emocionales o por situaciones del estrés propio del trabajo, eh. . . se, , hace un, se hace un poquito más eh, más eh, menos sensible a los problemas del paciente y es cuando el intérprete se da cuenta de que realmente lo que el paciente tiene es de extra importancia para que el médico no lo vea tan, tan importante. Creo yo que en estas situaciones tiende uno a favorecer un poquito más al paciente, puesto que uno es la voz del paciente. En muchas ocasiones sucede lo contrario, cuando el médico quiere hacerle preguntas que son cruciales para su diagnóstico final y el paciente responde con cosas que no vienen al caso, eh, desgraciadamente, mmm, mucho depende del nivel cultural del paciente, es cuando uno más o menos favorece al médico, nos vemos en la situación, hasta cierto punto estresante de no poderle comunicar, eh, la información que está pidiendo del paciente.*
>
> [There are situations when the doctor, due to excess of work, or emotional complications or work-related stress, becomes ehmm. . . less sensitive to the patient's problems. . . and it is in situations like these ones. . . when the interpreter realizes that the information the patient has is super important. . . and the doctor does not see it as so important. I believe it is in situations like this one, when one tends to side a little bit more with the patient, since one is the voice of the patient. In many cases it is the other way around, when the doctor wants to ask questions that are crucial for him to make a final diagnosis and the patient responds with irrelevant things. . . unfortunately, mmm, and this really depends on the cultural level of the patient. . and so in these cases, one more or less favors the doctor, we find ourselves in this. . . somewhat stressful situation of not being able to give the doctor, eh, the information that is being asked of the patient.]

When asked about the form of messages, the tone, body language, or even the channels through which interactions are interpreted, whether face-to-face, over the phone, videoteleconference and so forth, he acknowledges the role of his own experience by stating the following:

> *Ehmm, eh, fíjate que a pesar de que las interpretaciones son verbales y son por medio de teléfono, lo único que hemos perdido, muchas veces, son las caras que hace el paciente, eh, la forma en que gesticula lo que dice, este, se puede dar uno, un poquito más cuenta cuál es la gravedad de la situación o qué es lo que el paciente quiere decir. Muchos pacientes hablan con la mano, otros hablan con cambios faciales, y es lo que noto aquí otras veces que falta, al interpretar por. . . telefóno. Este, pero, obviamente, el caso de una interpretación por medio de teléfono, el tono de voz, no dice muchas cosas, eh, obviamente elevar la voz, el llorar, el decir, malas palabras a uno, se las dicen, no le dice al doctor, y no tiene que más o menos ser el réferi y decir, esto lo voy a decir, esto no lo debo de decir porque obviamente el médico se va a este, se va a molestar ¿verdad?, entonces, tienes tu propia experiencia como intérprete, te da la pauta para, para ser neutral hasta ciertos puntos, y, ser más enérgico, en otras situaciones, el paciente no te está tomando tanta atención tanto a ti como al médico ¿verdad?. . . por situaciones. . de que trae al chiquitín y/o la sobrina que viene con toda la familia.*
>
> [Hmm. . see, even when our interpreting is across spoken languages and done over the telephone, the only elements we may have lost are the patients' facial expressions. . . you know. . . the gestures patients make as they speak. . . these help one to. . . to grasp the severity of the situation. . . or the gestures help us realize what it is, really, that the patient wants to say. Many patients speak through their hands, others speak through facial gestures, and this is what we cannot see here as we do interpreting. . . over the telephone. . . Well, obviously when one interprets over the phone, the tone of the voice, does not say many things, uh, obviously raising the voice, crying, using bad words, they use bad words, I do not tell the doctor, and I have to be more or less the judge and decide: I'm going to say this, I should not say that, because obviously the doctor is going to. . . is going to be bothered right? Then, one has one's own experience as an interpreter. . . which gives one some guidelines for. . . to be neutral up to a certain point, and, to be more firm in other situations, if the patient is not paying as much attention to the interpreter or to the doctor, right?. . . and this is because they bring their little one and/or their niece, who also comes with her whole family.]

In addition, because interpreters are more familiar than providers with the cultural background of the patient, interpreters are in a position to understand, and even anticipate, culturally appropriate reactions on the part of the patient or even the patient's family members (see Chapter 7, excerpt from Julio's interview). In anticipating culturally appropriate reactions, they are contributing with their knowledge and their skills, which at times can enhance the quality of the interview. At the same time, if the anticipation is not contextualized, it may create misunderstandings during the interview. In the rest of this chapter, we focus on how interpreters deal with the content and form of messages which they interpret. The content of a message or a report, how such content is understood and discussed, depends on the background of the participants. In Chapter 3 we discussed how the provider, the patient and the interpreter may differ in their degree of expertise vis-à-vis medical/technical knowledge, cultural, linguistic and communicative knowledge as well as background knowledge of the issue triggering the encounter. In addition, the three parties vary in their degree of familiarity with the linguistic, cultural and social backgrounds of each and of the context in which the encounter takes place. Therefore, bearing in mind that message content and form are key to communication also means bearing in mind that we all differ in the way we access and construct information, which is discussed and transferred during communication.

Message content and form

Message content

In the particular case of healthcare, it is appropriate to differentiate between interpreters who work as freelancers in various community settings (e.g. in a hospital and also in a court of law, in a school or in a police interview) and medical/healthcare interpreters who are staff members, working full-time in a healthcare context. Interpreters who work as staff members in a healthcare context are immersed in a medical discourse community. They have a sense of belonging to the hospital culture. They have knowledge of the form in which things are said and asked. They are constantly exposed to ways of speaking of both parties for whom they interpret. They learn how patients and providers have different ways in which they ask and answer questions, they narrate or describe episodes or feelings, they explain or challenge statements and so forth.

From experience, interpreters learn that when the provider sets out to explore an answer, it is a different type of interaction than when providers ask for a yes/no answer. When providers need a yes/no answer to questions such as "Are you allergic to any medication?" or "Does it hurt or doesn't it?" (Angelelli 2001), providers go straight to the point, even if it means cornering the patient (Prince 1986). They need the answer to, for example, modify medication dosage or change a course of action (e.g. they may need to change currently prescribed treatment). Based on the information contained in an answer, providers make a diagnosis or a prognosis. Interpreters learn that in these situations, they will follow the provider's lead more than the patient's. If they do not have an opportunity to access interpreter education, to reflect on their practice, to learn about the responsibilities and roles of each of the participants, interpreters tend to repeat what they learn by doing. So, how can one get ready, how can one prepare? Interpreters crossing over to healthcare interpreting from other paths of life learn about ways of speaking by observing, interacting and listening to providers and patients in the course of doing their jobs.

As to the specific content of the assignments, healthcare interpreters learn to prepare for them by doing some of the following:

- Shadowing more experienced interpreters in the setting in which they work;
- Reading about the topic with which they need to work and analyzing the content;
- Gaining knowledge of the field in which they work (e.g. medical specialties, body systems, etc.);
- Learning new terminology by consulting existing glossaries or building their own;
- Doing parallel readings of an issue, a symptom, a procedure (using parallel materials in both languages with which they work);
- Accessing protocols in both languages (e.g. nurse or medical doctor protocols);
- Aligning texts electronically and building their own parallel corpus and glossaries.

As staff healthcare interpreters work in the same setting, they can benefit from taking notes on various types of encounters (e.g. make an appointment, receive results, undergo procedures) and learn some of the structure of the encounters as well as about the content and form of messages exchanged in them. They gain more information as they interpret the same or similar types of encounters, identify resources, shadow more senior interpreters, think about the types of medical encounters, explore reasons why patients go to the hospital, study protocols for procedures and anticipate issues. Staff healthcare interpreters have a clear advantage over freelancers in the sense that they are constantly building their knowledge on content and form of healthcare encounters.

Healthcare encounters are diverse. Access to hospital records may give us an indication of basic elements such as goals, duration and participants. Frequent and systematic observations over a prolonged period of time (such as the ones that result from ethnographies) give us details on the communicative event itself (its content and form). A seminal study on provider-patient interpreted communication conducted with Spanish-speaking patients and English-speaking providers over 22 months revealed the most frequent interactions in which the assistance of healthcare interpreters is required (Angelelli 2004: 71). In these interactions, interpreters worked face-to face as well as remotely:

- Schedule an appointment (mostly remotely)
- Place a phone call to cancel/change an appointment (remotely)
- Regular visit, check-up, follow-up (remotely and face-to-face)
- Explain condition/pain (remotely and face-to-face)

- Deliver news or results (remotely and face-to-face)
- Discuss treatment/plan of action (remotely and face-to-face)
- Hold educational sessions (e.g. on a condition such as diabetics, on nutrition for diabetics, or how to use a glucometer; pre-natal educational session for women suffering high blood pressure) (mostly face-to-face)
- Other issues (e.g. complain about a bill, attempt to locate a relative who has been hospitalized) (mostly remotely)

(Angelelli 2004: 71)

The study also showed that although some appointments are scheduled for specific purposes (e.g. to conduct a pap smear, give results, complete a presurgical visit, undergo surgery), one can never be 100 percent certain the unexpected will not happen (e.g. during a pap-smear test, the patient may start telling the nurse a story which contains relevant information about her medical history but that was never told before to the gynecologist) and different relevant information not anticipated will have to be interpreted. Thus there is a need for the healthcare interpreter to be flexible.

In addition, each of the types of encounters listed above may have a specific structure. A seminal study (Byrne and Long 1976) on behaviors of medical doctors in over 2,000 general-practice consultations identified the following six phases in GP encounters:

- Phase 1: relating to the patient
- Phase 2: discovering the reason for attendance
- Phase 3: conducting a verbal or a physical examination or both
- Phase 4: consideration of the patient's condition
- Phase 5: detailing treatment or further investigation
- Phase 6: terminating

The communication of content in each of those phases may be done in different ways (doctor may have more control, patient may deliver information in a different way than the provider would expect it, etc.). The way in which content is communicated (the form), in addition to how the presence of the interpreter interacts with the form, is discussed in the next session.

Message form

As we discussed above, in addition to content, messages have form. We study form by focusing on how a message is uttered by a participant and how it is delivered by the interpreter to the other participant. In the end, the other participant gets a blend of forms of the original utterance and the interpreted one. The interpreter may or may not be familiar with the ways of speaking of either the provider or the patient. The interpreter may or may not share a community of discourse with either of them. However, because one works for two parties, one needs to pay attention to the ways of speaking of both. This is an additional difficulty presented to the interpreter in healthcare encounters. In part this difficulty can be explained because, unlike other situations where interpreters work (e.g. a conference, a court hearing), in patient-provider encounters there is dialogue. The interpreter works in a mode that is referred to as dialogue interpreting (Cirillo and Niemants 2017). This means that the interpreter follows two parties (not just one) who are directly speaking to each other and interacting. When performing dialogue interpreting, the interpreter works into and out of the two languages. So, in addition to the element of dialogue and interaction, there is the element of language bi-directionality.

When interpreters work in conferences (e.g. a special conference organized by a well-known hardware company to launch a new product), the work is to interpret the speech of one speaker/signer (e.g. the keynote), in only one direction (language directionality), i.e. the language of some members of the audience with whom the speaker/signer has language in common. In this case, the speaker and the audience may or may not share the same language/culture associated to a country, region or language (and this is why they may need the help of a conference interpreter). They do, however, belong to the same speech community and share the culture of the hardware companies. Hardware developers/companies from the United States, Germany or Japan may not share the same language/culture (associated with a country, region or language), but they share a speech community: the one of hardware developers. So the conference interpreter, generally, does not have to juggle speech communities in addition to language and culture (associated to a country, region or language).

A healthcare encounter brings two parties who do not share a speech community (patients do not share the culture of the hospital, the ways of speaking of medical profession) in addition to not sharing language and culture (associated with a country, region or language). Therefore, for example, when a provider asks a patient about pain or about any other symptom discussed by the patient (temperature, nausea), the provider follows a protocol that is not shared by the patient (see Chapter 3). The provider needs specific information to make decisions. The patient hears the question and starts narrating, describing, telling a story. In these situations, interpreters need to coordinate the talk and the participation (Baraldi and Gavioli 2012) so that parties accomplish their communicative goals and needs within the allocated time. In addition to coordinating and managing at the macro level, interpreters also deal with coordination at the micro level.

With expertise in communication, interpreters know that the messages they deal with are not just made of words. They involve body language, gaze (Mason 2012), gestures and tone in addition to talking or signing. To add to this complexity, communication is governed by different rules in different languages. For example, while in Spanish two participants may speak at the same time (taking overlapping turns) – in fact they do most of the time, and this overlapping is considered the rule – in English they do not. In English, turn-taking (rather than overlapping) is the rule. So when patients and providers do not know that their languages differ at this level, they may pass judgment about each other and make assumptions that may not help communication. For example, if the provider is a user of a language that is based on turn-taking (e.g. English), the provider may think that the patient, a speaker of a language based on overlapping (e.g. Italian, Spanish' Turkish, among others), is impolite, as they are cutting into the conversation all the time, not letting the provider finish their sentences. Alternatively, the patient may wonder why the interpreter is asking them to wait, preventing them from speaking. Interpreters are able to coordinate talk at the macro and micro levels based on their knowledge about the ways of speaking and the communicative behaviors of the provider's and patient's discourse communities.

In addition to the complexity raising from juggling different languages, cultures, ways of speaking and discourse communities, doing all of this under pressure and in real time, interpreters also juggle working environments with different levels of technology. These differences require flexibility and adaptability on the part of interpreters as to how they approach their work. In the same day, a staff interpreter may work in a mental health ward, in which only face-to-face interpreting is used, and work remotely for providers, seeing patients in rooms or parts of the hospital wired for speakerphones, and for the reception counter where no speakerphone is installed (to observe privacy and confidentiality), and receptionist and patients pass a phone handle back and forth to communicate with each other with the assistance of the interpreter. Each of these situations presents specific challenges which may not be similar. In some public hospitals in the United States and Canada, some private fertilization clinics in Greece or private hospitals in Spain, especially attracting medical tourism (Angelelli 2015) staff interpreters may also work remotely with video. So, while they are still working remotely, the fact that there are portable computers with cameras standing in providers' offices or wheeled to a hospitalized patient's room allows for video calls. This helps the interpreter have eye contact, be part of the interaction and still not be physically present.

As discussed in the literature on remote interpreting (Braun 2015), work done remotely presents advantages and disadvantages. Specifically from staff-healthcare interpreters, participating in research studies, we learn that remote interpreting allows them to work from one spot (rather than walking from appointment to appointment across a main hospital and/or the surrounding clinics). In addition, the physical distance from the interaction affords interpreters more detachment from difficult situations (e.g. disconnecting patients from life support in front of family members, breaking bad news) (Angelelli 2004, 2015). On the other hand, working remotely requires interpreters to pay even more attention to tone, pauses and so forth, and rely on the provider-patient to guide them through visual cues that the interpreter cannot see (e.g. providers may verbalize the steps they are taking during a neurological exam and the patient's response, because interpreters cannot see the interaction between provider and patient). In this case, providers learn how to guide interpreters and interpreters working remotely learn how to be guided. The upside for healthcare organizations is that using remote interpreting increases productivity and many times patients' satisfaction (as they do not have long waiting times). The downside for interpreters is that remote interpreting affords them less downtime or fewer breaks. In sum, the way in which interpreting is conducted impacts both content and form of the interpreter's rendition. We now will briefly discuss one of the most challenging specialties in which healthcare interpreters work.

Content and form in mental health encounters

The rising prevalence of mental illness is a growing concern for many societies, and access to mental health care is one of the top public health priorities. In addition, as more and more people migrate and settle or take refuge in countries with a dominant language other than their own, the need for interpreting/cultural mediation in mental health care settings is also on the increase. Interpreting for mental health patients presents specific challenges for the interpreter. The most important one is that, unlike most interpreting communicative events, in which interpreters may pay unequal attention to content and form, negotiate understanding and many times produce text not given to them (Angelelli 2004: 78), for mental health providers, form and content are key elements, so interpreters need to resist doing what many times they do (e.g. editorializing, toning down). Patients may not be of sound mind to express what they need to express, and providers need to examine the form in which something is expressed (the language used and the content produced by patients), without any editorializing on the part of the interpreter.

Therefore, in the specific case of healthcare interpreting in mental health, interpreters need to rethink their goal. In this particular case, they need to help the provider extract data from the client and render it "as is" in the target language, paying attention to both content and form and trying to preserve them as intact as they possibly can. They do this because they understand the difference between verbatim and trying to bridge communication, trying to help or broker. They need to do their work as if they were interpreting in a court of law. In fact, in mental wards, many times interpreters find themselves working between a patient, a provider and an officer of the court. The dynamics of a healthcare encounter are changed and made more complex by the addition and the presence of a third party to the interaction: the interpreter (Angelelli 2004).

Given that mental health is a more challenging setting, one should ask what is unique about a mental health encounter and what changes occur in the psychotherapeutic setting when an interpreter brokers communication. The mental health context presents specific issues (Bot 2006). These issues are impacted by the presence of an interpreter mediating the interaction (Miller et al. 2005). One of these particularities is the need for establishing a therapeutic working alliance (Bordin 1979). A brief review of the literature on interpreting in mental health settings reveals several guidelines aimed at mental health care providers working with interpreters (Amodeo et al. 1997; Tribe & Thompson 2011; Tribe and Tunariu 2009; Judd et al. 2009). They highlight the additional ethical responsibilities of providers as a result of including an interpreter in the setting (Wright 2014).

The addition of an interpreter changes the dyadic mental health relationship into a triadic one (Tribe and Morrissey 2004). This statement is frequently found, although the specifics of the changes have not been explored in depth. We do not really know if/how the changes in a mental health encounter are different from the changes in any other type of healthcare encounter caused by the addition of a third person. Studies focusing on interpreters in mental health settings are limited in quantity and methodology. Most studies report on interviews conducted with clinicians who discuss their experiences. The limited availability of empirical data poses a problem and raises more questions than it provides answers. For example, Miller et al. (2005) explored communication in a mental health setting by interviewing 15 interpreters and 15 healthcare providers regarding their therapy work with refugees. They concluded that the presence of an interpreter does affect the therapeutic relationship and that there may exist an added complication in the form of transference and countertransference processes between the three participants. They also noted regular reports by clinicians stating that (1) the construction of the therapeutic alliance in interpreted-mediated encounters was more gradual than in "standard" monolingual encounters and (2) interpreter-patient trust was seemingly established *before* patient-therapist trust. This latter finding is echoed in Pugh and Vetere (2009), who interviewed ten mental health professionals with interpreters in the therapeutic setting. The focus of the interviews was empathy construction. The authors reached similar conclusions to previous studies showing that the practitioners interviewed were concerned because of the change in the empathy dynamics arising from working in a triad. In addition, they expressed some uneasiness as they explained that sometimes the interpreter would not render the "empathy" they wished to communicate. Empathy is a crucial component of the psychotherapeutic alliance, necessary for therapy to succeed (Pugh and Vetere 2009).

The concept of "therapeutic equivalence" was used by Bot (2005) to bring together interpreting theory and Hill's typology of therapeutic actions to account for the cases in which interpreters render information correctly, but not therapeutic intent. This is particularly relevant for our discussion on content and form of messages and the competing goals of all interlocutors (see above and discussion in Chapter 3). There have been calls for specific training of interpreters working in mental health to avoid these issues (see, e.g., Bot 2005; Pugh and Vetere 2009). In addition, a collaborative model for working with interpreters (Raval 2005, 2006) refers to the figure of the interpreter as a "bilingual co-worker" to the mental health provider. This approach is characterized by clearly defining the interpreter's role in a pre-session meeting and by strong collaborative dynamics with therapists including training interpreters within the therapeutic institution. Working with deaf patients and building on their experiences of using sign language interpreters in psychotherapy, Bruin and Brugmans (2006) also emphasize the need to establish a therapist-interpreter working alliance in order for the therapy to succeed. They also discuss the importance of defining the interpreters' role clearly and jointly (in collaboration with therapists) prior to the session.

It is important to note that, in studies in psychotherapy involving interpreter-mediated interactions, the trust on the interpreter is also discussed from the patient's point of view and findings are similar. If the patient mistrusts the interpreter, this may inhibit discussion and patient disclosure. However, once again, studies are mostly experiential and they do not discuss how/if trust gets built with the interpreter in the first place. In cases of refugee patients, for example, they may mistrust the interpreter if they perceive them as coming from an "enemy" ethnic group or having a different political viewpoint (Miller et al. 2005: 32; Amodeo et al. 1997). Similarly, if both interpreter and patient are from a small language community, this may lead to mistrust and confidentiality concerns on the part of the patient (Tribe and Thompson 2011). This echoes findings from studies with asylum seekers in general and users of less commonly spoken languages coming from small, tight communities or rural areas.

The interpreter's gender is also extremely relevant in certain therapeutic treatments, and many researchers stress that this should be taken into account when selecting an interpreter (Tribe and Lane 2009; Tribe and Tunariu 2009, Amodeo et al. 1997; Raval 2005; Hsieh et al. 2013). This is also the case in other healthcare specialties (e.g. obstetrics and gynecology, transgender presurgical appointments). Issues of therapy effectiveness were examined in an experimental study (Schultz et al. 2006) in 53 refugee patients who were suffering from post-traumatic stress disorder (PTSD). One patient group was treated in the patient's language by a bilingual practitioner while the rest received treatment using interpreters. The study found a high degree of therapy effectiveness in both groups examined. The effects on refugee interpreters working in therapy with refugees suffering from trauma have also been examined (Engstrom et al. 2010; Miller et al. 2005, Green et al. 2012). Researchers concluded that the patients' memories and stories could trigger strong emotional reactions including strong transference and countertransference reactions (Miller et al. 2005). Interpreters' own trauma histories (Green et al. 2012) could also be retriggered by their work and exposure to similar issues. Miller et al. (2005) state that the benefits of working with refugee interpreters (shared stories which lead to better degrees of trust and empathy) outweigh the issues presented, but that interpreters should work on these cases only if they have made significant advances on their own trauma recovery and if they have a strong social support network, otherwise the risks may overwhelm them. Engstrom et al. (2010) and Green et al. (2012) advocated for institutional support for the interpreters in addition to training interpreters in self-care techniques (Green et al. 2012).

The need for debriefing session is identified as key to help interpreters process problematic emotional-content sessions (Tribe and Thompson 2011; Raval 2006). There is, however, a warning to this practice, as it may trigger an ethical conflict (Wright 2014). As the therapist treats the interpreter, a multiple relationship may develop. This multiple relationship between the patient, the provider and the interpreter may contradict ethical standards and generate confusion on part of the therapist as to whom (i.e. the interpreter or the patient) is indeed the client/patient in the therapeutic treatment. Given this potential conflict, it is recommended that interpreters be overseen by a different therapist than the one they regularly work with, or that the interpreting agency itself provide those services to their interpreters. Control of the session flow is also an issue examined in the literature. Participants in some of these studies (Pugh and Vetere 2009) expressed concern over the interpreter's control of the turn-taking. However, other studies (e.g. Zimányi 2013) yield contradicting findings while exploring the same issue through a series of interviews, concluding that both therapist and interpreter share control of the session, and that while interpreters take control of the information flow, ultimate control of the session rests with the mental health professional. Bot (2005) also examined this issue. She states that the model of interpreting used (interpreted as translation machine versus an interactive model of interpreting) affects session control, and noted that when the interpreter is handed too much control of the session, this may lead to problems. She also advocates a collaborative model where practitioners are aware of the complexities of introducing an interpreter in the interactions and actively work to tackle the known risks.

B. Research, observe and reflect

Exercise 1: openings and closings of interpreted communicative events

In this exercise we look at one opening and one closing of an interpreted communicative event. As you read the example, pay attention to what the interpreter does with language (content and form). Think of the consequences of openings and closings of the interpreted communicative event.

Example 1: opening

The interaction takes place at Lavender Clinic. It is an urgent care clinic close to the main hospital in town. Mary is a nurse working at the clinic. Mr. Lopez has been waiting patiently for over two hours. When he is called by the nurse, as he follows the nurse he starts telling the nurse how difficult it has been to get an appointment with the doctor and how he has been missing days of work waiting and he wants to be seen and x-rayed today. The nurse calls the main hospital language service unit to get an interpreter on the line. Irene, the Spanish/English interpreter, is assigned to work in this call. The nurse briefs Irene on the phone and tells her what the patient has said (she does not understand Spanish).

As you read, reflect on what Irene does on turn 2 and 4.

1 N Please tell him that we need to know why he is here and we do not speak Spanish, that is why you are here!
2 I Okay Mary. Let me first introduce myself to the patient. *Muy Buenos días señor Lopez. Me llamo Irene y le voy a ayudar a comunicarse con la enferemera Mary de la clínica Lavender Field.*
Good morning Mr. Lopez. My name is Irene and I will help you communicate with Mary, who is the nurse at Lavender Field Clinic.
3 P *Muy agradecido. . . pero mire. . . este oiga. . . hace tiempo que me tienen esperando. . . que el doctor no está. . . mire que me dan vueltas. . . que necesito que me miren el pie. . . que tantito estaba mejor. . . pero que desde que me calce otra vez. . . es que. . .*
I appreciate it, but, see, it has been too long. . . I have been waiting to get an appointment for too long. . . the doctor is not in?. . . I have been given the run around. . . I need someone to take a look at my foot. . . it was doing better before. . . but I started wearing shoes again. . . and. . .
4 I *Sí, sí señor comprendo. . . ahorita le dice a la enfermera. Espéreme, un momentito. . .*
We are ready Mary.
5 N Okay, so ask him what is the main reason for coming to see us today.

What does the transcript tell us about how Irene positions herself? Discuss her politeness, her empathy, her responsibility and so forth. Is Irene interpreting in lines 2 and 4? Were lines given to her? Or is she using her own initiative to coordinate the talk? To claim her place in the interaction? What does she accomplish in turn 4?

And now we look at the closing of the same interpreted communicative event.

Example 2: closing

35 N Okay, that's all then, thanks.
36 I Okay Mary. Thank you. *Gracias señor Lopez, que tenga buen día y Buena suerte!*
Thank you, Mr. Lopez. Have a good day and good luck to you.
37 P *A usted. Muchas gracias, muy agradecido, eh. . .*
38 I Bye.
39 N Bye.

What does Irene do in line 36? Why does she do it? Who closes the interaction with whom? With these reflections in mind, depending on your access to medical encounters, study openings and closings involving your two (or more) working languages. Whether you can access encounters yourself or you can look at data already published by others, whether the encounters take place face-to-face or remotely, take notes to transcribe and reflect on how interpreters handle the content and form of the message as they do their work.

Exercise 2: interpreter coordinating talk remotely

The following is a segment of a transcript of an authentic doctor/interpreter/patient interaction (Angelelli 2001). We will focus on the content and the form of communication. The patient is visiting the eye doctor at California Hope, a public hospital in California (Angelelli 2004). The reason for his visit today is that, based on the previous test results, the patient is considered glaucoma suspect. The eye doctor wants to find out if there is a history of glaucoma in the patient's family and conduct further tests. The previous results were within the limit. The patient and the doctor are face-to-face. The patient speaks Spanish and the eye doctor speaks English. The interpreter is joining remotely. A speakerphone in the room allows both patient and doctor to hear the interpreter's voice without passing a telephone handset back and forth to each other. This is the typical arrangement in this public hospital. Both patients and providers are used to this three-party communication and, although the interpreter is a staff member of the hospital and works on site, he is not in the same room where the visit is taking place. Once the doctor calls the language service unit in the hospital and requests an interpreter, the interpreter joins the interaction via a speakerphone (the hospital is wired for this type of communication). The patient is reporting itching in both eyes. The patient believes this itching is connected to his vitamin or medication intake. We join the conversation after the doctor has introduced himself, explained to the interpreter from which clinic he is calling, and after the interpreter has introduced himself to the patient, explored the patient's background and concern, as guided by the eye doctor. This background information will help us contextualize the segment, as we join the interaction in turn 54.

Read the transcript carefully and then answer the questions at the end.

54 I He is saying that he has a problem with his eyes he has itching in both eyes and that's been going on for about two years and last year in Mexico he went to a doctor. The doctor told him that he may have allergies
55 D Uh-huh
56 I The patient is saying that he notices that every time he takes vitamins
57 D Uh-huh
58 I Or any medicine he says he has itching eyes
59 D Okay well so he's not taking any medicine now?
60 I *Señor ¿Está usted tomando alguna medicina?*
Sir, are you taking any medicine?
61 P *Ahorita no*
62 I No medicine
63 D So he is not having itching now?
64 I *¿Le queman los ojos estos días que no está tomado medicina?*
Are your eyes itching these days when you are not taking medicine?
65 P *Hmm. . . apenas tengo. . . la semana pasada me terminé un frasco de vitamina*
Hmmm. . . I just. . . last week I finished a bottle of vitamins
66 I He is saying that last week he finished a container of vitamins and yes he started itching eyes

67 D Okay well what did. . . he's already using artificial tears he can add to that another over the counter umm medicine for allergies like that's it's called Naph-cona

68 I Okay can you spell it doctor?

69 D I'll write it out for him N A P H the dash C O N A. It's over the counter. I'll hand this to him.

70 I *Dice la doctora le va dar escrito en un papel el nombre de una medicina que va a comprar sin receta*
The doctor says she will write for you on a piece of paper the name of a medicine that you can buy over the counter

71 P Okay

72 I What about the artificial tears? Is he going to buy it over the counter?

73 D Yes he's already. . . he's already he is already using those

74 I *Okay dice que siga usando las eh lágrimas artificiales*
Okay. . . She says you should continue to use the hmmm artificial tears

75 P *Sí*

76 I *Y además de eso ella le va a dar una receta de una medicina nueva que usted va a comprar sin receta*
And she's also going to prescribe for you a new medicine that you're going to buy over the counter

77 D And if the Naph-cona is inadequate he can come back to the clinic and there is something stronger we can prescribe

78 I *Y si esta nueva medicina que le da ella escrita en un papel que se llama Naf-cona sino es suficientemente efectiva usted debe volver y le van a dar otra. . .*
And if this new medicine that she wrote on a piece of paper for you called Naf-con is not effective enough, you should come back and you will be given another one

79 P *Okay pero ¿son gotas pa* [sic] *los ojos?*

80 I This Naph-cona are they drops doctor?

81 D Yes uh-huh

82 I *Sí son gotas*
Yes, they are eye drops

83 P Ah okay

84 D Okay umm so that's it. They will be contacting him about when his visual field is

85 I *So entonces el hospital se va comunicar con usted para darle otra cita para hacerle otro examen de los campos visuales*
Okay then the hospital will communicate with you to give you another appointment for another examination of the visual fields

86 P Okay

87 I *¿Tiene usted algo que preguntar?*
Do you have any questions?

88 P *Es todo*
That's all

89 I *¿Eh?*

90 P *Es todo gracias*
That's all, thank you

91 I No questions
92 D Okay thank you very much
93 I Thank you doctor
94 D Alright bye
95 I Bye

Reflecting on this transcript that results from empirical research, focus on the following questions:

Focus on content. What is this encounter about? What can you say about the content of the interaction?

a Identify medical (technical) terms. List five of them.
b Do you know what they mean? Give synonyms or paraphrase them.
c Can you define glaucoma?

Write different ways in which you can explain glaucoma if the patient you work for is (1) a young educated adult; (2) a child accompanied by a parent; (3) an older patient who refers to parts of the human body as animal parts, indicating a lower level of education.

Focus on form:

a What is the interpreter doing in turn 64? What does he want to achieve by adding "that you are not taking any medicine"?
b What is the interpreter doing in turn 68? Why is he requesting this from the doctor? This line was not given to the interpreter by either the provider or the patient. Is this interpreting? Is this enabling communication? Are these two the same thing?
c What do you see happening in the shaded area (turns 68 to 83). Is this interpreting? Is it coordinating? Is it the same? Would you do this if you were interpreting face-to-face?
d What does the interpreter do in turn 87? This line was not given to him. Why is the interpreter doing this? Do you have enough context to answer? Do you think a staff interpreter and a freelancer would react in the same way? If yes/no, how can you explain your answer?
e How does this interaction close? What would you have done differently?

C. Journal writing

Based on the concepts discussed in this chapter, the transcript presented above (section B), and your work on the answers to the questions and the exercises in Further Tasks (section C), reflect on what your work as interpreter entails. To do this, think of your work as divided in three different parts/stages:

1 Before the assignment
2 During the assignment
3 After the assignment.

In your journal entry for this chapter, discuss what you have learned about content and form in each of these stages, what you can do at each about content and form both for the assignment at hand and for future assignments. Have you thought about interpreting/communication in this way before? Is understanding and analyzing messages at the level of content and form new to you, or do you do this regularly? If so, do you see the benefit of transferring these skills to your work? If not, why? Do you think it is feasible? If not, why? Have your views about interpreting changed? If so, how?

D. Further tasks

Exercise

This is an example of a nurse protocol. Please read and after reading proceed to the questions below.

Select appropriate care advice (CA)

- Give care advice for those patients who don't need to be seen or who will be seen later by appointment. See rationale, "When Less is Better," below.
- Make sure the caller has a pen and paper handy to write down instructions. This is especially important if detailed care advice or medication dosages are given.
- The nurse should select the most appropriate 2–3 pieces of care advice for the caller. The nurse should not feel compelled to give all the care advice.
- Complete care advice is displayed for patients that can be seen by appointment or can be cared for at home. However, consider it a "menu" from which the nurse delivers "a la carte."
- Some callers may benefit from 3–6 pieces of information; others may only need 1 or 2 pieces. The triage nurse should select care advice as determined by the caller's needs.
- Try to limit your advice to 3 instructions and try to keep your comments brief (2 or 3 sentences per instruction). Reason: to improve caller's memory of imparted information.

(Cleartriage 2018)

After reading the protocol, please think about the following questions and draft some answers:

1. What is the purpose of having protocols?
2. Who designs the protocols? Who uses them?
3. What happens if protocols are changed in content? Give an example of a change to protocol content.
4. What happens if protocols are changed in form? Give an example of a change to protocol form.
5. What can we, as HIs, learn from using the already existing protocols written for providers with whom we will be interpreting?
6. Are protocols universal?

Exercise: fact or myth? (eye contact, looking at floor)

Here are some statements we may hear about healthcare interpreting. Based on your observations, readings, knowledge of the field and experience in it, decide if they are facts or myths. Your decision should not be based on your opinion, rather on a fact that you can point at and show to others.

Statement	*Fact? Myth?*	*Justification*
The interpreter should manage the communication flow during the encounter and keep both parties informed about it.		
When interpreting remotely, interpreters should request the provider to do things they cannot do remotely or cannot see as done (e.g. give the patient the name of a referral specialist, or a telephone number discussed in writing; give the patient a copy of the presurgical instructions just discussed in the language of the patient, if available).		
The interpreter should seek clarification before rendering statements.		
The interpreter should ask the participants to speak in short sentences.		
The interpreter should sit behind the patient to be able to whisper discreetly.		
The interpreter can only work with words.		
The interpreter should remind the parties not to speak at the same time.		
The interpreter should always open and close the interactions for the others and for the self.		
While interpreting face-to-face, interpreters should avoid eye contact with the participants by looking at the floor. This will encourage eye contact between the provider and patient.		

Exercise: anticipating content and form in medical encounters

In this exercise we focus on specific medical issues. We brainstorm what we anticipate could be the content discussed and we also write down the forms in which the content/issue may be discussed, the reactions of participants and so forth. In the following table, there are some types of encounters HIs work on regularly. Give some thought to what is discussed and how it is discussed by both patient and provider. Fill the table with the information you have. Then think about how you, as the interpreter in these sessions, would prepare to work with the content and form that will come up in the medical encounter to which you are assigned. Also make a list of things that you believe may not be anticipated.

Type of encounter	*Message content (what?) and form (how?) one can anticipate*
Diabetic education session	– Content: – Form:
Regular visit, check-up, follow-up	– Content: – Form:
Place a phone call to cancel/change an appointment	– Content: – Form:
Deliver news or results	– Content: – Form:
Discuss treatment/plan of action	– Content: – Form:
Explain condition/pain	– Content: – Form:

Message content	*What can one anticipate about message form (how?) from the participants? How would they react to and talk about this content?*
Breaking bad news: The biopsy is positive for breast cancer currently at stage 3. It is a very aggressive type.	– Patient – Provider
Exam results imply the patient has not been taking his medication as indicated. Patient instead has been donating the prescribed medication to his church. Provider is baffled by the lying and expresses his frustration to the patient. Tension is high.	– Patient – Provider
End of life decision: It has been six months since the patient was put on life support. There having been no change, the medical team advises to withdraw support.	– Patient – Provider

References

Angelelli, C. V. (2018). Cross-border healthcare for all EU residents? Linguistic access in the European Union. *The Journal of Applied Linguistics and Professional Practice*, 11(2), 113–134.

Angelelli, C. V. (2015). *A study on public service translation in cross-border healthcare technical report*. Luxembourg: Publications Office of the European Union. ISBN 978-92-79-47163-6.

———. (2012). Challenges in interpreters' coordination of the construction of pain. In C. Baraldi & L. Gavioli (Eds.), *Coordinating participation in dialogue interpreting* (pp. 244–260). Amsterdam: John Benjamins.

———. (2004). *Medical interpreting and cross-cultural communication*. London: Cambridge University Press.

———. (2001). *Deconstructing the invisible interpreter: A critical study of the interpersonal role of the interpreter in a cross-cultural/linguistic communicative event.* PhD dissertation, Stanford University, Stanford, CA.

Amodeo, M., Grigg-Saito, D., & Robb, N. (1997). Working with foreign language interpreters: Guidelines for substance abuse clinicians and human service practitioners. *Alcoholism Treatment Quarterly, 15*(4), 75–87.

Baraldi, C., & Gavioli, L. (Eds.). (2012). *Coordinating participation in dialogue interpreting.* Amsterdam: John Benjamins.

Bordin, E. S. (1979). The generalizability of the psychoanalytic concept of the therapeutic alliance. *Psychotherapy: Theory, Research and Practice, 16*(3).

Bot, H. (2006). Community interpreting in mental health: Research issues. *Linguistica Antverpiensa, 5.*

———. (2005). *Dialogue interpreting in mental health.* Amsterdam and New York: Rodopi Publishers.

Braun, S. (2015). Remote interpreting. In H. Mikkelson & R. Jourdenais (Eds.), *Routledge handbook of interpreting* (pp. 352–367). New York: Routledge.

Bruin, E., & Brugmans, P. (2006). The psychotherapist and the sign language interpreter. *Journal of Deaf Studies and Deaf Education, 11*(3), 360–368.

Byrne, P. S., & Long, B.E.L. (1976). *Doctors talking to patients: A study of the verbal behaviours of doctors in the consultation.* London: HMSO.

Cirillo, L., & Niemants, N. (Eds.). (2017). *Teaching dialogue interpreting.* Amsterdam and Philadelphia: John Benjamins.

Cleartriage. (2018). Available at www.cleartriage.com/wp-content/uploads/STCC-OH-Users-Guide (Last accessed June 2, 2018).

Engstrom, D. W., Roth, T., & Hollis, J. (2010). The use of interpreters by torture treatment providers. *Journal of Ethnic & Cultural Diversity in Social Work: Innovation in Theory, Research and Practice, 19*(1), 54–72.

Green, H., Sperlinger, D., & Carlswell, K. (2012). Too close to home? Experiences of Kurdish refugee interpreters working in UK mental health services. *Journal of Mental Health, 21*(3).

Hsieh, E., Pitaloka, D., & Johnson, A. (2013). Bilingual Health Communication: Distinctive needs of providers from five specialties. *Health Communication, 28*, 557–567.

Judd, T., Capetillo, D., Carrion-Baralt, J., et al. (2009). Professional considerations for improving the neuropsychological evaluation of Hispanics: A national academy of neuropsychology education paper. *Archives of Clinical Neuropsychology, 24.*

Mason, I. (2012). Gaze, positioning and identity in interpreter-mediated dialogues. In C. Baraldi & L. Gavioli (Eds.), *Coordinating participation in dialogue interpreting* (pp. 177–200). Amsterdam: John Benjamins.

Miller, K. E., Martell, Z. L., Pazdirek, L., Caruth, M., & Lopez, D. (2005). The role of interpreters in psychotherapy with refugees: An exploratory study. *American Journal of Orthopsychiatry, 75*(1).

Prince, C. (1986). *Hablando con el doctor: Communication problems between doctors and their Spanish-speaking patients.* Ph.D. diss., Stanford University, Stanford, CA.

Pugh, M. A., Vetere, A. (2009). Lost in translation: An interpretative phenomenological analysis of mental health professionals' experiences of empathy in clinical work with an interpreter. *Psychology and Psychotherapy: Theory, Research and Practice, 82.*

Raval, H. (2006). Mental health training for bilingual co-workers in the context of working with people seeking asylum and refuge. *Primary Care Mental Health, 4*: 37–44

———. (2005). Being heard and understood in the context of seeking asylum and refuge: Communicating with the help of bilingual co-workers. *Clinical Child Psychology and Psychiatry*, *5*, 541–562.

Schultz, P. M., Resick, P. A., Huber, L. C., & Griffin, M. G. (2006). The effectiveness of cognitive processing therapy for PTSD with refugees in a community setting. *Cognitive and Behavioral Practice*, *13*, 322–331.

Tribe, R., & Lane, P. (2009). Working with interpreters across language and culture in mental health. *Journal of Mental Health*, *18*(3): 233–241.

Tribe, R., & Morrissey, J. (2004). Good practice issues in working with interpreters in mental health. *Intervention*, *2*(2), 129–142.

Tribe, R., & Thompson, K. (2011). Developing guidelines on working with interpreters in mental health: Opening up an international dialogue? *International Journal of Culture and Mental Health*, 4(2), 81–90.

Tribe, R., & Tunariu, A. (2009). Mind your language: Working with interpreters in healthcare settings and therapeutic encounters. *Sexual and Relationship Therapy*, *24*(1), 74–84.

Wright, C. (2014). Ethical issues and potential solutions surrounding the use of spoken language interpreters in psychology. *Ethics & Behavior*, *24*(3), 215–228.

Zimányi, K. (2013). "Somebody has to be in charge of a session": On the control of communication in interpreter-mediated mental health encounters. *Translation and Interpreting Studies*, *8*(1), 94–111.

Further readings

Cornes, A.,& Napier, J. (2005). Challenges of mental health interpreting when working with deaf patients. *Australas Psychiatry*, *13*(4). pp. 403–-407.

Crezee, I.H.M. (2013). *Introduction to healthcare for interpreters and translators*. Amsterdam and Philadelphia: John Benjamins.

Drew, P., & Heritage, J. (Eds.). (1992). *Talk at work: Interaction in institutional settings*. Cambridge UK: Cambridge University Press.

Nadeau, L., Rousseau, C., & Measham, T. (2014). Addressing cultural diversity through collaborative care. In L. J. Kirmayer et al. (Eds.), *Cultural consultation: Encountering the other in mental health care*. New York: Springer-Verlag.

Tribe, R., & Raval, H. (Eds.). (2003). *Working with interpreters in mental health*. Brunner-Routledge: Hove and New York.

5 Skills and competencies

Receptive skills

With Christian Degueldre

GOALS

In this chapter we will:

- Understand the importance of the skills involved in interpreting.
- Familiarize ourselves with the receptive skills and competencies involved in healthcare interpreting.
- Focus on the receptive skills for interpreting (command of both languages, active listening, text/discourse analysis).
- Reflect on the skills and competencies involved in interpreting in general and healthcare interpreting in particular.
- Become familiar with acquiring, developing and self-assessing the necessary knowledge and skills to become a healthcare interpreter.

LEARNING OUTCOMES

By successfully completing this chapter, we will be able to:

- Learn about the preparation of an assignment.
- Identify useful and less useful materials for practice.
- Discriminate between ways of speaking and terms.
- Differentiate between listening and active listening.
- Learn about anticipation.
- Pay attention to content and form.
- Improve skills through exercises, practice, observation, analysis and reflection.
- Gain experience in guided self-reflective practice.

This chapter and the next one are about the skills and competencies that interpreters in general and healthcare interpreters in particular use while interpreting. This chapter focuses on the preparation for an assignment and on receptive skills. Chapter 6 deals with productive skills. In both chapters, we want the reader to understand what is involved in each skill and to learn how to practice. We achieve this first through guided self-reflective practice. After working together, we suggest activities that can be repeated in order to improve each particular skill. Therefore, the structure of Chapters 5 and 6 differs from the other chapters, as the activities are spread throughout, rather than presented in specific sections (as in sections B and C). As in previous chapters, the reader is invited to do some personal reflection in the form of journal writing. After the references, in the Further Readings section, the reader will find supporting materials to further learning and practice of the skills we describe as well as others used in interpreting in general.

A. Competencies and skills

What are the competencies and skills that healthcare interpreters (HIs) exhibit? Are they the same as, similar to or different from those generally found in court or conference interpreters? What specific skills do interpreters need to interpret in a healthcare setting?

Definitions

Sometimes, the terms "skill" and "competence" are used as synonyms, and indeed they are not. We will define them first to avoid confusion. Dictionaries may contribute to this confusion by defining "competency" as "an ability or skill" in its version for English language learners (Merriam Webster 2018).

Interpreting between a nurse/doctor/healthcare professional and a patient is a competency. To effectively interpret in a medical setting, one needs to have good analytical, interpersonal, interpretive, linguistic, logical and socio-cultural ability. This means one must be highly proficient in both the source and the target languages, be sensitive to the culture of both parties, be able to take notes, use one's memory effectively, listen actively, show empathy and so forth. All of these are skills.

"A competency is the capability to apply or use a set of related knowledge, skills, and abilities required to successfully perform 'critical work functions' or tasks in a defined work setting" (Council on Linkages Between Academia and Public Health Practice 2012).

In a healthcare-related setting, **competency** "utilizes appropriate methods for interacting sensitively, effectively, and professionally with persons from diverse cultural, socioeconomic, educational, racial, ethnic and professional backgrounds, and persons of all ages and lifestyle preferences" (Council on Linkages Between Academia and Public Health Practice 2012).

A **skill** is defined as a "sufficiency of qualification; capacity to deal adequately with a subject." It is "the capability of accomplishing something with precision and certainty; practical knowledge in combination with ability; cleverness, expertness. Also, an ability to perform a function acquired or learnt with practice" (OED 2018).

In the above definition of skill, the notion of "qualification" appears. As in any profession, for an interpreter being "qualified" is a crucial element that contributes to their "professionalization" and better "recognition" (see Chapter 1).

Interpreting a patient-provider encounter

In an interpreted patient-provider encounter, the three co-participants come together to accomplish a goal, and because they do not share a language, the patient, the provider (doctors, nurses, social workers, lab technicians), and the healthcare interpreter need to work together for a positive health outcome for the patient. This is referred to as the healthcare team. Each member of the team brings specific skills. Research on provider-patient communication has identified some of the contributions expected from provider and patient during an encounter.

Communication between patients and providers: examples of contributions

Expected contributions from patients (AAOS 2013):

- Participate in decisions about own healthcare. Research shows that patients who take part in decisions about their healthcare are more likely to have better outcomes.
- Educate yourself about your condition.
- Ask your doctor to give you easy-to-read brochures or other patient-friendly literature so you can learn about your diagnosis, medical tests and treatment. Make sure you understand everything. If you don't understand something, keep asking questions until you do.
- Speak up and ask questions.
- Your doctor and healthcare team want to understand your questions and concerns.
- Ask for help from an advocate.
- Consider involving a trusted family member or friend in your care.
- Know the medications you take.
- Medication errors (i.e. wrong medication, wrong dosage) are the most common healthcare mistakes.
- Know your healthcare providers.
- Take time to learn about the doctor, team and hospital providing your care.

Expected contributions from providers (Ranjan et al. 2015):

> The process of curing a patient requires a holistic approach, which involves considerations beyond treating a disease. It warrants several skills in a doctor along with technical expertise. Studies have shown that good communication skill in a doctor improve patient's compliance and overall satisfaction. There are certain basic principles of practicing good communication. Patient listening, empathy, and paying attention to the paraverbal and nonverbal components of the communication are the important ones that are frequently neglected. Proper information about the nature, course and prognosis of the disease is as important.

To find out what skills the interpreter needs to bring to the encounter, we imagine the following scenario: you are a freelance medical interpreter. You have been asked to interpret next week during a medical appointment at the local clinic. The patient is a 50-year-old woman with limited English proficiency and shares your native language. She has been diagnosed with diabetes and needs to talk to her clinician about the treatment, her overall health and nutrition in general.

Activity: skills associated with the stages of interpreting

As the interpreter, make a list of all the things you will need to do before, during and after the assignment, using the table below. As you may think of many tasks (actions) that you may need to do during the medical interview, add space as needed. For each stage/activity, think of the skills that are associated with this activity. Focus on the skills that you need to use (develop further) in order to perform the different tasks.

Actions/tasks	*Associated skills*
Stage 1: Before the assignment	
If possible, I should find out the case/area of healthcare and try to get as much information as possible about the goals for the assignment.	Preparation and research skills as part of the inquiry process
I need to read about the topic (disease, diagnosis, test, procedure, etc.) because I am not familiar with it.	Research (conceptual and terminological) Anticipation of content and form of the assignment Topics to be discussed; terms to be used How patient and provider may talk about the topics How patient and provider may handle questions, answers, complaints, bad news, etc. about the topic
. . .	. . .
During the assignment	
Pay attention to what the parties say to each other.	Active listening Concentration
Pay attention to how parties talk/sign and interact with each other. Pay attention to body language, tone, gestures.	Multitasking: listen to what is expressed, observe how it is expressed, react to how it is expressed
Be sensitive to the way concepts are uttered. . . is the patient upset?	Sensitivity to tone, body language, gestures, gaze
. . .	. . .
After the assignment	
Update my knowledge of topic/type of encounter.	Organize terms and ways of speaking – preparing for next encounter
. . .	. . .

Compare your list of actions/tasks with the following list of tasks. These tasks have been identified as necessary for a healthcare interpreter to be effective (Angelelli and Degueldre 2002: 84). Then, think of all the items you have that are not in the following list and the ones you may not have included and reflect on their relative importance.

At the listening stage

Ability to comprehend form and content
Ability to identify accent, regional variety and register
Ability to listen carefully (content and details)
Ability to follow a message at normal speed with very little/too much repetition
Ability to perceive tone
Ability to exhibit empathetic listening/understanding.

At the information processing stage

Ability to anticipate information by following the structure of the talk
Ability to understand the meaning of a message (content and form)
Ability to ask for clarification
Ability to politely signal/interrupt to alert parties of a misunderstanding/ issue that may arise
Ability to formulate responses/questions
Ability to switch between one's language register and that of the speaker/signer
Ability to switch between one's language dialect and that of the speaker/signer
Ability to switch between one's way of speaking/signing and that of the speaker/signer
Ability to understand instructions and sequencing of events

At the delivery stage

Ability to adapt to varieties of language (geographical, social)
Ability to adapt to how each participant talks/signs and uses language
Ability to produce a message at normal speed, without unnecessary repetitions or with deletion of relevant information
Ability to use communicative strategies (rephrase, describe, illustrate) in a transparent way
Ability to produce oral language at a near-native level, in a socio-culturally appropriate way (including, among others, register, tone, vocabulary, grammar)
Ability to produce messages empathetically
Ability to paraphrase technical terms/explain concepts in lay terms, if requested/required
Ability to produce instructions and sequence events
Ability to perceive body language feedback from speakers and act accordingly (repeat, clarify) in a transparent way

Importance of communication

Before dissecting the skills involved in interpreting, we should remind ourselves that communication lies at the base of interpreting. The problem with all forms of communication, including interpreted ones, is that breakdowns might occur at different points. Even when we share a language, in communication there is no guarantee that the receiver decodes the sender's message in the way it was intended. In the case of interpreting, breakdowns can occur in the course of reception of the message, its analysis or its reproduction. The ability to communicate effectively with the healthcare provider and the patient(s) remotely or face-to-face is crucial. It helps the patients, who are assured that the healthcare provider fully understands their needs; it helps the healthcare provider in delivering the best possible care. And most importantly, effective communication allows all parties involved to act in the best interests of the patient. Healthcare interpreting puts the user of the non-societal language who seeks access to healthcare virtually on an equal footing as a speaker of the societal language.

Receptive skills

The skills presented in this chapter are related to some of the following competencies: linguistic competence, interpreting competence, research, technical competence, "interpersonal competence" and socio-cultural competence.

As discussed at the beginning of this chapter, we divide the competencies and skills in two parts: those associated with the reception of the message and those associated with the production of it. This chapter focuses on the reception skills – mainly those associated with the linguistic competence and those linked to interpreting competence. In Chapter 6, we will focus on the productive skills.

Skills associated with linguistic competence

Linguistic competence (i.e. being competent to understand and use the language in its various registers, varieties and forms) is basic for interpreting. In fact, one cannot interpret what one does not understand. In the context of interpreting, linguistic competence refers to the ability to comprehend the source language and render the message in the target language. It means that the interpreter must be able to understand and use technical and non-technical language at different levels of formality. Speakers have different accents, socio-economic backgrounds and registers and may use formal, informal or colloquial language and idiomatic expressions. Having linguistic competence allows the interpreter to understand and produce messages in a socio-culturally appropriate way.

In-depth knowledge and understanding of languages

Whether one interprets for providers, administrators or patients in a hospital, mastering the language of both parties is a prerequisite to performing. In a medical setting, this means not only focusing on the terminology but also in the ways in which each of these parties speak about issues (see Chapter 3), paying special attention to body language, gestures, the nuances of the message and the implied meaning (implicature). The interpreter must understand different accents. Needless to say, the interpreter is expected to have appropriate vocabulary, grammar, intonation, pronunciation, body language, gestures, socio-cultural awareness, range of registers and fluency in both languages. The use of the language cannot constitute an obstacle to communication between patient and healthcare provider.

Ability to shift language registers and ways of speaking

Healthcare providers and patients not only do not speak the same language but, equally important, they do not share the same register or speak in the same way about a topic. They belong to different speech communities (see Chapter 3). Being able to understand the way a doctor speaks and the way a patient speaks (and what each is able to understand from the other) calls for the interpreter to understand and/or use a wide range of registers and ways of speaking. This will ensure successful communication.

Skills associated with interpreting competence

Interpreting is "communicating." To communicate effectively, the interpreter must understand the communicative goals of patient and provider: what the patient and the healthcare provider say, and how they say it (See Chapter 4). That implies a good knowledge of the topic that will be covered during the encounter. The interpreter is required to prepare thoroughly.

Preparation – knowledge of subject area

Familiarity with a topic allows the interpreter (or any listener for that matter) to understand what is being said. For example, if one has to interpret for a consultation with an ophthalmologist about a possible cataract surgery, one reads about the anatomy of the eye, about cataracts, about the current procedures to treat them and so forth. One may even read about the physics of light reflection and the function of the retina. Any of these topics may come up in various levels of detail during the encounter. There are numerous resources to research a medical issue such as cataracts. The interpreter is responsible for reading and gaining knowledge on topics to understand what experts say about the topic. In this way, interpreters can interpret from speakers who belong to a different speech community (i.e. experts in ophthalmology) than the interpreter (Angelelli 2000).

It is important to think big but start small. This means that in preparation for this encounter, one first reads some introductory books on the topic. These are usually written in simpler language, which is necessary to understand more advanced concepts. Once one establishes a base knowledge, one can move to the next level to access more difficult information. Jumping directly to a more complex type of text, one for specialists in the topic, may prove unsuccessful. One simply does not have the background knowledge of a given discourse community (the one of experts in ophthalmology) to access it without background. One may not understand the concepts well and may ultimately be discouraged.

Information abounds, so one cannot claim ignorance. Discriminating between genuine and non-genuine information is a skill we also have to develop. Interpreters look for information in various sources that are published for different readers. Some pharmaceutical companies, for example, offer a plethora of information on their websites that can be helpful to interpreters because they cater to different readers. They are meant for clients (who are not experts). The MSD Manuals (2018) are written at two levels: a consumer version for patients, parents or caregivers and a professional version for medical professionals or students. They are published in different languages (Chinese, English, French, German, Italian, Japanese, Portuguese and Russian). When comparing a text written in two languages, if they are translations, one must first make sure that the translation can be trusted and is produced by a reputable party.

Active listening

"Listening is the activity of paying attention to what speakers say while trying to work out what they mean" (Underwood 1989). What is active listening? In conflict resolution, "active listening is a way of listening and responding to another person that improves mutual understanding" (Burgess 2013). Often when people talk to each other, they do not listen attentively. They may be distracted, half listening and half thinking about something else. They assume that they have heard what the other person is saying; rather than paying attention to what is said, they focus on how they can respond to win the argument.

Every day we get a lot of information by listening to the voices around us: family members, friends, the news on the radio and television, messages on social media or information from coworkers. A child learns a language by listening to all the sounds around her. We are familiar with what we hear in our own house, we are used to the noises and we may become nervous when we hear new noises in a new place.

Listening is a very important part of our daily life. It is very often done automatically. Most of the time, we do not pay close attention when we listen. Listening is an important skill for interpreters. Interpreters cannot listen in the way just described, as they will miss important information. Interpreters are expected to state the complete content of the message in the target language. To do that, they need to listen in a different way than they regularly do in their daily lives. Interpreters acquire a special way of listening. They learn to listen actively. To be effective in any communication, and especially in health and mental health settings, the interpreters need to be active listeners. Healthcare providers (i.e. doctors, nurses, social workers and psychologists), all members of the healthcare team – interpreters included – need to develop good active-listening skills.

Active listening is a structured form of listening and responding. It puts all the attention on the speaker. To do this, the listener focuses on the speaker and the message. This allows the listener to then restate what the speaker said. Active listening is a skill that requires practice. Following are some tips on becoming an active listener.

SELECTION OF MATERIAL FOR ACTIVE LISTENING

Selecting a suitable material for practice is not an easy task. Very often we find that some texts/speeches are too difficult, too slow, too dense, not challenging enough and so forth. In addition, it is important to pay attention to the content of the message but also to its presentation and style, to the ways in which speakers/signers produce messages.

We should consider the following to evaluate suitable material to practice active listening:

Content	
Select a familiar topic	It will allow you to focus on listening, not on understanding and making sense of new information.
Avoid technical topic	A technical topic, with challenging terms and concepts, may make you focus on the trees and miss the forest.
Choose a topic in your mother tongue first	Although you can do this exercise in any of your working languages, you will find it easier at first to listen in your mother tongue.
Avoid any unnecessary challenges on the part of the speaker	Avoid speakers with a heavy accent. Avoid multiple speakers at a time, which makes it more difficult to follow one.
Define the context	Understanding is more feasible if one is already aware of the context. That allows for the activation of the right schemata.

Style/presentation	
Type of texts	There are various types of texts: persuasive, performative, instructive and descriptive (Reiss 1989).
Register	Is the text formal/informal? Does it contain slang? Have you noticed register shifts (switching between formal and informal) in the text you have selected?
Intonation	How is intonation used? For what purpose?
Pronunciation	Are speakers/signers easy to understand?
Length of segment	Do not start with a long message. . . three or four minutes might be already very challenging at the beginning. It is always possible to use longer segments later, once we have become more familiar with the exercise and have gained confidence.
Explicit and implicit message	Was the message always explicitly stated, or did you have to guess what was implicit in it?
Speed of delivery	Choose a speed which is comfortable: a delivery that is too fast will create an unnecessary difficulty at the beginning of practice; the same holds true for an unusually slow delivery.
Read texts	Avoid messages read as they don't usually provide the same natural pauses, hesitations and repetitions that you would find in natural speech/signing. For this reason, prefer spontaneous interviews to prepared remarks or the daily news on your TV set.
Background noise	If you are using recorded input, avoid segments with background noise, at least at the beginning. It is difficult enough to actively listen to one voice in a clear environment.

(*Continued*)

(Continued)

Abusive use of proper names	A proper name is difficult in the sense that it does not have an intrinsic meaning. Avoid texts with long lists of names (e.g. attendee lists).
Abusive use of figures	Figures usually do not mean much by themselves. Avoid texts with isolated figures (e.g. math exercises).

As we improve our active listening skills and become more confident, it may be good to increase the difficulty of the materials (denser, longer, with heavier accents, on a less familiar topic, etc.).

After learning how to select an appropriate segment/program for listening, let us apply what we have learned using an audio segment. Please record a radio program, an internet program, a podcast, a TED Talk or the news on your favorite radio station. Listen carefully to the recording. Then proceed to evaluate it using the Practice Sheet for Text Selection, below.

ACTIVITY: TEXT SELECTION

Use the audio below to assess a text, then check with our suggestion.
Universal health coverage in Rwanda (World Health Organization – WHO)
www.youtube.com/watch?v=GmQiA4J-XDw&feature=youtube

Practice sheet for text selection

Content	
Select a familiar topic	Dr. Olushayo Olu, from World Healthcare Organization in Rwanda, describes the work of WHO to support the government in providing a community-based health insurance scheme for people working in the informal sector.
Avoid technical topic	Not very technical.
Choose a topic in your mother tongue	English (segment with English subtitles).
Avoid any unnecessary challenges on the part of the speaker	No repetition. Only one speaker.
Define the context	Given the economic situation, not many people have health insurance in Rwanda.

Style/presentation	
Type of text/speech	Statement on community-based health insurance, very factual
Register	Familiar
Intonation	Normal
Pronunciation	Slightly difficult accent from Rwanda (Africa)
Length of segment	2'16"
Explicit and implicit message	No implicit message – very factual
Speed of delivery	Normal, sometimes slow – didactic
Read texts	No read passage
Background noise	None

Abusive use of proper names	No – just the local name in African language, Ubudehe
Abusive use of figures	No
Abusive use of acronyms	No

Comments on this material: the topic, although not entirely familiar, is a topic of interest to many people. It is presented in a way that does not require a specific knowledge or an advanced terminology. The speed of delivery is adequate. The text does not present any particular challenge except for the accent of the speaker. It is not very long and deals with one single topic.

SUGGESTIONS FOR SOURCES OF MATERIALS AND RECOMMENDATIONS FOR PRACTICE

There are many sources we can use for practice: a radio program discussing a topic of interest in your area (e.g. public transportation), an interview on TV, a documentary on the internet (on your favorite radio or TV program) or a discussion between a patient and a nurse during a medical encounter (you can use published transcripts and ask a friend to record those for you). We provide some links at the end of this chapter to sources and materials you can use. You should expand the list with your own references and favorite sites. After identifying appropriate sources (oral/video signed texts) for practice, we focus on how we can use them to improve our active-listening skills.

The following are only a few suggestions of how we listen, for what purposes and so forth. As always, feel free to add to these ones your own. We can listen to a text (1) for its content (when we are looking for information only); (2) for its form (to see how text is presented; how the form in which messages are stated may impact the listener); and (3) for language (as a pedagogical tool for language learning; you will then pay more attention to grammar, intonation, terminology, etc.). We start with *Listening for Content:*

Before listening once (only) to the segment below, paying special attention to its content, ask yourself a few questions such as:

1 What is the main idea of the passage you have just heard? Try to explain this in one or possibly two short sentences. Imagine you are telling this to a friend who has not heard the information.
2 What are the supporting elements or supporting ideas? Answer this question by trying to explain what you just heard with more information.
3 What are some of the key words used? Stating key words will help you get to a more detailed level of understanding the text.
4 Are all the elements of meaning presented explicitly? If not, which elements are implicit, left to your deduction and analysis? Are you able to discover the implicit message? When discussing content, you may ask yourself questions not simply about what has been said (the explicit part of the message) but also the implicit elements that you can only discover if you are able to listen carefully and attentively to tone and so forth, doing what is called reading between the lines.

First main idea	
Supporting idea	
Key words	
More. . .	

PRACTICE SHEET ON LISTENING SKILLS

Use this Practice Sheet on Listening Skills to determine what are the main ideas, the supporting ideas and some key words used in the following segment, then compare with our suggestions.

Listen once (only) to the interview segment below, paying special attention to its content. The interview is on stress. Follow this link: https://healthradio.fm/interviews and look for the interview of Jean-Paul Gravel on stress from 2015–11–10 (Healthradio 2018). If the reader cannot find this audio on the internet, a recording is provided on the Routledge website at www.routledge.com/9781138232952.

Now that you have listened to the text and marked the Practice Sheet, you may check with our suggestion below.

In our example:

First main idea	*Stress and mental illness*
Supporting idea Key words More. . .	National day to make us aware of stress Deal with stress, dissolve it
Second main idea	*Why are we stressed and what to do about it?*
Supporting idea Key words More. . .	Signs of mental illness and stress Physical and emotional stress, sleep, digestion, depression, anger

Repeat for each new main idea

Third main idea	*Firsthand experience with stress*
Supporting idea Key words More. . .	It was a nice case study Depression, anger

Etc. . .

Fourth main idea	*Through conversation*
Supporting idea Key words More. . .	You are not broken Training for healthy life; unhealthy belief
Fifth main idea	*Etc. . .*
Supporting idea Key words More. . .	Etc. . . Etc. . .

Listening for style Using the same recording, ask yourself a few questions.

What is the purpose of the text/speech? Is it a letter from school to *inform* the parent about an upcoming event? A manual that *instructs* you how to use a new appliance? A political figure in your community who tries to *persuade* you to vote for them? A story that *describes* life in Lapland?

What are the different methods used to get the message across to the listener?

Persuasive texts might use: repeated words text in capital letters exclamation marks rhetorical questions (questions where no answer is needed) an emotional one-sided argument humor a convincing tone	**Informative texts usually:** avoid repetition contain facts give information in a clear way – introducing the subject and then developing it
Instructive texts: are written as though the reader is being spoken to – (although the word "you" is not usually used) the language is direct and unnecessary words are left out often use "must" and "must not" sometimes use diagrams or pictures to help understanding	**Descriptive texts usually:** make use of adjectives and adverbs use comparisons to help picture it – something is like something employ your five senses – how it feels, smells, looks, sounds and tastes

Knowing the type of text/message you are dealing with will help you find the right "way/tone/form" to interpret it. You may ask yourself: are there many repetitions in the message? Are those repetitions intentional? What is the purpose of the repetitions and how is that purpose achieved?

According to how you answer these questions, you may decide to skip some repetitions or to interpret every single one of them.

Listening for language Now use the Practice Sheet on Listening Skills to determine the type of language used, whether it is formal or familiar, assess the register, the use of slang and so forth.

In our example:

Purpose of text	*Typical informative text*
Methods used	No repetition Contains facts Gives information in a clear way – introducing the subject and then developing it. Progresses in a clear, structured way.
Repetitions/intentional	Main ideas presented as titles are expanded with facts
Register shifts	Factual information with no register shift
Use of slang	None
Use of synonyms	None
More. . .	

You may repeat the exercise focusing on intonation, register, terminology and so forth. Listening is a skill that is improved through guided and reflective practice.

You may practice using the Practice Sheets for Text Selection and Listening Skills with any other texts of your choice.

Text/discourse analysis

As we have discussed previously in this book, communication implies understanding. In order to understand, one must analyze the discourse and reflect on how a message is constructed, produced, processed and received. Even when messages (oral or written) are considered text, there is a difference in how translation and interpreting conceptualize meaning and its transfer. As we discuss text analysis, it is important to remind ourselves of this difference. Otherwise we may fall into the trap which states that the difference between translation and interpreting is that the former deals with written texts and the latter with oral ones. While this is true, another important difference is that in translation there is a text and its meaning can be construed and interpreted differently by readers or translators. The reader is alone in accessing it and does not co-construct meaning with any other party. To translate a message, translators deal with a text, have to understand its content and form properly, its context, its time, analyze the (hidden) meaning and restate it in the target language in a socio-culturally appropriate way (adapted from Bassnett 1991). Healthcare interpreters instead deal with communication (rather than information transfer only) and meaning is co-constructed and negotiated by all the participants in the interaction (including the interpreter) in real time. Healthcare interpreting conceptualizes communication as human interaction rather than information transfer.

By analyzing the message/text, by processing the information received, we understand it better and we can render its meaning. Analyzing text (oral or written) is like putting what we say or what we hear under the microscope. Let's consider an example of a provider-patient interview in which the nurse is asking the patient about medicine intake. The nurse speaks clearly; her questions are short and she tries to obtain only the information she needs in specific answers. The patient answers telling a story, with digressions, giving examples. When the nurse or the patient speaks, we could ask ourselves a few questions that will shed a different light on the meaning exchanges. The answers to these questions may be different for each participant. For example:

- Is the message straightforward? The nurse's yes, the patient's not so much.
- Is it dense and complex? The nurse's no, the patient's story may be convoluted.
- Are there repetitions of the same idea or not? Yes, and this may be for different reasons for each of the parties.
- Are the ideas explained? The nurse may explain them briefly and clearly. The patient may attempt to explain them through a story and may be cut off, redirected to the initial question, etc.

Further questions that guide analysis could be more general or more specific. Read the examples of questions below and decide if they are general (at the macro level) or specific (at micro level), and now it is your turn to answer them.

- What is the goal of the provider or the patient?
- Is the content presented in a logical way, or is it presented in an unstructured, not so clear way?
- Does the listener need to have prior knowledge of the topic in order to understand the message, or is it self-explanatory?
- Are there difficult terms, which are key to understanding?
- Does the message contain idiomatic expressions, jargon or domain-specific terms?
- Do the speakers use images, metaphors or straight language?
- Do the speakers use repetitions, paraphrasing and other linguistic tools to express ideas?

The goal of analyzing a message (a statement made by the provider, a question asked by the patient, an answer, a description of a procedure, a narration of a daily routine) is to find clues that will help us understand it better. It is similar to the work of a detective. Some of the clues are outside the text/message itself – we call them extratextual factors as opposed to the intratextual factors, which are factors relating to the text itself, including its nonverbal elements.

What does this mean? In the example of the interaction between a patient and a nurse on medicine intake discussed above, we once again use Hymes's framework of ethnography of communication (Chapter 3) to see what elements we identify before and during the interaction.

Extratextual elements	
Who	Sender of the message: nurse
What for	Nurse needs information about medicine intake
To whom	Recipient: patient
How	Talk and labels from medications that patient brought in a bag
Where	Clinic – Nurse's office/San Diego, US
When	Wednesday 11:00 a.m.
Why	The patient is going to start taking a new medication and the nurse needs to verify the current medicine intake to make sure medication is all compatible
Intratextual elements	
What	Content of the nurse/patient encounter; emerged from the interaction during the appointment
What not	Knowledge the nurse supposes that the patient has; knowledge the patient has and assumes the nurse knows
In what order	The order in which content is presented; aligned with a typical protocol for medicine intake or different
How	Way of speaking about content; form of the content in the interaction

The elements presented in the first table above (extratextual elements) generally precede the interaction during the medical encounter. In our example, the healthcare interpreter may be told (some non-confidential information is included in the scheduling of the assignment) who the parties that need interpreting are (the nurse's full title, what area they work in, etc.; what information is available about the patient), what the medical issue is that will be discussed and so forth.

Anticipation

We start with some definitions of anticipation.

Anticipation is a process of co-relation among factors pertaining to the present, past and future of a system (cf. Nadin 2018).

> The act of anticipating, taking up, placing, or considering something beforehand, or before the proper time in natural order.
>
> Previous view or impression of what is to happen; instinctive prevision; foretaste; as, the anticipation of the joys of heaven.

Interpreters generally note that it is easier to interpret a topic with which they are familiar than a completely new topic. You can experience this when you interpret for a patient/provider whom you already know instead of interpreting for a patient or provider you have not met before. This is because you already know more or less what to expect: you know the topic, you have heard the person speak/saw the person sign, you know the context, thus your level of anxiety is lower. You know that interpreting is easier when you know or can guess what the speaker (doctor/patient) is going to say next. You are able to determine this, to anticipate because you have prepared the topic well, you know what to expect and also because you are able to put your knowledge and preparation to good use during the doctor/patient encounter. All of this allows you to anticipate rather accurately what is coming next.

As the interpreter identifies with the parties for whom they interpret, they follow the trend of thought and are able even to anticipate mentally what the next part of a sentence or sometimes of a message is going to be. That helps them confirm that what they hear next is actually what was to be expected. In this case, the interpreter simply compares the message with the expected outcome. The ability to anticipate can be learned and taught. It is also a way to verify that the interpreter is "tuned" with the parties for whom they interpret.

If we go back to the quote, we see that anticipation implies a co-relation between past, present and future. As we interpret, we use our previous knowledge (the past) to understand a present statement by the doctor or a patient, as we already think about the potential implications that that has for the future of the encounter and we already anticipate the reaction of the other party.

For interpreters (and translators), the past is everything: they have read about a medical topic, it is the exposure they have had to medical encounters, the experience of having heard particular accents, the familiarity with the ways in which providers and patients speak, all the experience we have accumulated over the years of interpreting at the clinic or at the hospital, it is our discussions with our colleagues about difficult terms or phrases. It is, in other words, our general (and specific) knowledge of the domain and the situation which allows us to better understand the ways patients talk about what happens to them and/or the recommendation that doctors give to patients. And as we are listening to what a patient is telling the doctor (this is the present), we are probably also thinking about what is going on in the doctor's mind as a result as well as what their reaction might be. We try to anticipate the future turns of the encounter. But, as we do this, we are very careful! We need to listen to what is said rather than to what we think (or anticipate) will be said.

Anticipation is useful when we communicate with someone directly or when we interpret to help two people (e.g. a doctor and a patient) talk to each other. Anticipation allows us to guess what the answer to a question will be. If we are not sure we understand the question or the answer, we can ask the person to say it in other words (clarification of information, rephrasing). This is why anticipation is important in the education of interpreters. However, we must be careful not to fall in the pit of the last definition of anticipation: hasty notion, intuitive preconception. If we do, we will commit the error of not listening properly and jumping to conclusions. We cannot impose what we think we understand onto what was said.

In our preparation for an interpreting assignment, it is important to warm up and think about the content of – and the terms that may be used in – that assignment. As you can see, thinking about what might happen during a specific medical encounter is also one way to anticipate. Let us suppose the next assignment is about smoking, the danger of smoking and so forth.

ACTIVITY: SMOKING: AN ADDICTION

You look at your schedule for the coming week. In four days you are going to interpret for Dr. Brown, a general practitioner for whom you have interpreted before, and Bill, a teenage patient. He is a chain smoker and will come to see Dr. Brown about his addiction. You want to prepare yourself as much as possible, and for this you will do some research and preparatory readings. You had never interpreted any encounter related to smoking, but you know the harms of smoking and several of your friends are smokers.

To warm up and start activating your knowledge on smoking, make a list of topics and terms that are related to smoking. Think about them in your language combination.

Terms about smoking, statistics about smoking, the danger of smoking, etc. in the societal language	*How would I say them in my other language?*

In anticipation of the assignment we should also think about (1) what the patient might tell the physician and (2) what the physician might tell the patient.

Use the following space to write down your list of terms that you think will be used by each participant as they talk. When you have finished, check with the list below, which comes from observing this interview (Angelelli 2001).

What the patient (Bill) might say	*What the physician (Dr. Brown) might say*

Let us check with parts of the provider-patient interview transcript:

Some of the things Bill said:
"I used to be able to run a mile under six minutes. Now I'm lucky to make it in nine. And I'm wheezing all the way." "Until recently, I smoked two packs a day. Now I am down to ten cigarettes. I want to quit. But it's not that easy." "A lot of my friends smoke. I feel smoking helps me being part of the group. I do not like to be pointed out as the weird guy because I do not smoke like most of my friends do. Plus I am with my friends all the time and I know I will continue to get secondhand smoking even if I quit. Isn't that worse?" "Even though I know smoking is not good for me, it seems I cannot stop. . . What can I do?"
Some of the things Dr. Brown said:
"Ok, Bill, many teen smokers quit; many keep some of the old friends and many make new ones." "Teen smoking rates have steadily fallen, but the numbers are still too high." "I am not trying to scare you, Bill, but to help you realize how serious an addiction nicotine is." "That's more than 1 million teens a year. Roughly one-third of them will die from a smoking-related illness." "There are different programs to help young people stop smoking." "Teens have a choice: they can become victims, or they can stop before they go too far. Better yet, they never have to start at all." "I can recommend some help groups."

Based on our readings of protocols, as general practitioners also talk about the dangers of smoking and addiction in general, we can anticipate that Dr. Brown may explain how smoking affects someone's health and provide some statistics.

ACTIVITY: BEST EXERCISE FOR MORBIDLY OBESE PEOPLE TO LOSE WEIGHT (RAY 2017) AT WWW.LIVESTRONG.COM/ARTICLE/274887-BEST-EXERCISE-FOR-MORBIDLY-OBESE-PEOPLE-TO-LOSE-WEIGHT/

1 Using the following table, make a list of ideas and terms (in English) that you believe will be used in talking about weight loss, obesity and diet-related topics.

English terms about diet and exercise, etc.	*How would I say this in my other language*

2 Then proceed to analyze the following short text and write your answers to the questions that apply to this text.

Best exercise for morbidly obese people to lose weight

Obesity is a serious health condition that can lead to diabetes, heart disease and other medical complications. The Highland Hospital Bariatric Surgery Center defines morbid obesity as having a body mass index of over 40 or being over 100 pounds overweight. Minor weight loss can begin to reduce the effects of obesity and lead to healthier benefits. In addition to a balanced, low-calorie diet, you must include physical activity to lose weight. The morbidly obese should start slowly on an exercise plan and increase the time and intensity of workouts as they gain strength.

Identification

Many people who are morbidly obese have medical conditions and disabilities that require physician monitoring. According to the American College of Sports Medicine, if you are morbidly obese, you should undergo a stress test to identify your current level of fitness prior to starting an exercise regimen. A stress test can help your doctor determine a base level from which you should begin to prevent injuries and overexertion that could lead to further complications.

Features

Anyone who has not exercised in a while or who begins a new exercise program will feel some discomfort. Muscles that haven't been used can become painful when engaged. An appropriate exercise for the morbidly obese may include some discomfort but should not create significant lasting pain. Muscle reaction typically is delayed and felt the day following exercise. Any physical activity that causes pain while you are doing it and continues the next day should be stopped and reported to your doctor.

Extratextual factors		*Write your answer here*
Who	Author of the text	
What for	Sender's intention	
To whom	Recipient/addressee	
How	Medium or channel	
Where	Place	
When	Time (text is written or read)	
Why	Motive	
Intratextual factors		
What	Subject matter, information presented in the text	
What not	Knowledge the author supposes that the reader has	
In what order	How is the text presented	
How	Words used, grammar, intonation	

3 Using the list of terms you have created in English and the information from the text itself, make a list of terms in your other language.
4 Using the list of terms in your other language and what you remember from the original text, make a speech in your other language.
5 Find information related to the topic at hand on the internet and complete your glossary of terms in English and the other language.

B. Research, observe and reflect

Now that we have discussed the various skills used by interpreters, let us critically reflect on what this means for us at our own level. The following are examples of some skills. The lists of areas/questions can be used as a self-checking guide to raise our awareness on what we do well, what we need to focus more on and what we need to learn. Through guided self-reflection, you may design a personalized learning plan reflecting your needs.

Preparation – knowledge of subject area

- What are the healthcare/medical resources in your area that can be useful to learn specific terminology?
- How can I improve my medical knowledge and thus my understanding of medical issues?
- How can I become more familiar with patients' and providers' ways of speaking about medical issues?
- How can I understand the language used by the patient and the healthcare provider?

You can read information and build your bi/multilingual glossaries by visiting the websites of international organizations, which provide documentation in different languages (World Health Organization, United Nations, European Union). This example for French illustrates what you can do for other languages: Société Européenne de Médecine de Sapeurs-Pompiers (Comité français) Protocoles Infirmiers de Soins d'Urgence Version 2014 / 2015, www.infirmiersapeurpompier.com/tinymcefilemanager/file/2015-07-07_17-19-05_referentiel_pisu_semps.pdf contains a list of emergency nursing protocols (*protocoles infirmiers de soins d'urgence*). This could be how one could start a tailor-made bilingual French-English glossary.

You may look at the various professional associations (nurses, psychiatrists, ophthalmologists, etc.) in your language combination in various areas where your languages are used (to incorporate regional ways of speaking and varieties) and at the international level. In the example given, we could explore resources in French from Belgium, Canada, France, Senegal and so forth.

Linguistic skills and register

An interpreter needs to keep up with two languages and its many varieties and discourse communities. Interpreters are constantly searching for ways to improve their linguistic skills not only in their second/heritage language but also in their first language if they live in an area that does not use it. Although experiencing full exposure to a second language (live in an area where the language is spoken) is always advisable, it is not the only way in which linguistic skills can be enhanced.

In addition to taking a course abroad, one can also take courses, training sessions, observe professionals in their daily work (as in internships), read books and newspapers, take part in specific healthcare interpreting or communication chatrooms, in special-interest groups interacting in one's second language, read blogs, listen to podcasts, TED talks, and watch medical shows on television or YouTube channels. In our global village, technology has made access and exposure to other languages and cultures more feasible than ever, so we can do all of the above from one portable device wherever we are.

Here are some things one can do to enhance language and register:

Make a list of what you read. Think of the respective value of all your readings. Ask yourself these questions: Why am I reading this? Am I reading for information, for language, for fun?

Look up readings that are quite different from the ones you read. Decide on a topic first (e.g. appendicitis, bulimia, sudden infant death syndrome). Look for readings on the health-related topic of your choice that target different segments of readers. For example, if you choose bulimia, look for (1) a reading a specialist would use (e.g. a research paper reporting on an experimental treatment for the condition); (2) a reading from a popular science magazine (which explains scientific issues in a simple way for the lay person to access them); and (3) an article from a popular press (i.e. targeting sixth grade readers), in which a pop star may be telling their own journey on this issue or may have been interviewed about it. This variety of readings can help you get examples of different registers and ways of speaking about the same topic.

Make a list of the radio or TV programs you enjoy. Look for some that present not simply the news but also discussions, unrehearsed impromptu exchanges with people calling in to the station. This will expose you to different accents and different registers. You may notice it is sometimes easier to understand the news than people in the street.

Look for websites that present healthcare/medical news, such as the World Health Organization, the Pan-American Health Organization and MedlinePlus of the US National Library of Medicine (US National Library of Medicine MedlinePlus 2018). Use these forums to pay attention to the language used, the register, the slang, the terminology, the accents and the intonation.

Active listening

Activity 1: individual practice

Write down ten things you remember listening to this week.

For example: *I listened to the radio this morning.*

1 ______________________________
2 ______________________________
3 ______________________________
4 ______________________________
5 ______________________________
6 ______________________________
7 ______________________________
8 ______________________________
9 ______________________________
10 ______________________________

Now, write down what you remember from those ten listening experiences, trying to include as many details as possible.

Activity 2: pair practice

For this activity, you need a peer/colleague to do this with you. In your first or second language, write three full sentences that describe your morning routine. Work in pairs and take turns playing the roles of the speaker and the listener. The speaker will tell the listener the information about the daily routine (not read verbatim, rather as giving information). When the speaker stops, the listener will repeat what the listener thinks the speaker said. This allows the speaker to find out whether the listener really understood. If the information is not correct, if the listener did not understand or forgot, the speaker will restate the information again. After the listener is able to restate the information correctly, the activity will be repeated with a change of roles: the listener becomes the speaker.

Building active listening takes time, reflection and practice. There are many opportunities each day to practice active listening. You can ask friends or family members to help you practice this same activity.

To begin choose material that is not highly technical or complex. If something is too technical, one may be tempted to worry about the words. In so doing, one may miss what the other person is saying (the meaning of the message). It is best to start doing this activity in the language that you are most comfortable; then repeat the same activity in your other language(s).

Activity 3

Continue working with a partner. One of you creates a story that may be based on an article from the newspaper or heard on the radio and presents it orally. The other one listens to the story that is presented.

Then the "listener" answers the following questions:

> What is the "point" of the story? What does the writer want you to remember about this story? The point of the story is called the *main idea.*
>
> ___
>
> Write down the *main idea* of the story in two or three short sentences.
>
> ___
>
> ___
>
> ___
>
> Summarize the main idea into one sentence that conveys as much as possible about the whole story.
>
> ___
>
> ___
>
> Thinking again about the story, what are the details that helped you "see" (have a mental representation/image) what was described?
>
> ___
>
> ___
>
> ___
>
> What are some of the key (important) words that were used?
>
> ___
>
> Are there any emotions that the writer tries to make you feel?
>
> ___
>
> Now repeat the same activity with a different short story in the other language of your language combination; the listener from the previous activity becomes the speaker. The same steps will be used to discuss the story.

What is the "point" of the story? What does the writer want you to remember about this story? The point of the story is called the *main idea*. Use one or two words.

____

Write down the *main idea* of the story in two or three short sentences.

____

____

____

Summarize the main idea into one sentence that says as much as possible about the whole story.

____

____

____

Thinking again about the story, what are the details that helped you "see" what was described?

____

____

____

What were some of the key (important) words that are used?

____

Are there any emotions that the writer tries to make you feel?

____

C. Journal writing

Having compared your list of skills to the one suggested at the beginning of this chapter, you may note similarities and differences. Take a moment to reflect on the importance of the skills you did not think of when you were doing the exercise. Ask yourself some questions. For example, what are the necessary steps in my preparation for interpreting at a medical encounter? How am I going to organize technical terminology? How am I going to classify ways of speaking? How can I keep my glossaries up to date? Shall I keep a log and bookmark the best internet sites, articles, books I found? How am I going to make room in my schedule to practice the various skills I have learned in this chapter?

D. Further tasks

Other exercises associated with enhancing active listening

John Murphy (1991) suggests various exercises to improve listening in the language classroom. You may also practice your active listening skill using other exercises such as the following:

- Silent reading while listening to audio material

Many programs on the internet are available in MP3 or WAV file formats and are accompanied by the transcript of the program. You may perform a silent reading of the transcript as you listen. This will make you more aware of the basic qualities of the spoken material: its speed, use of intonation, use of specific terminology, pronunciation and so forth. It is also a good exercise to check understanding. As you check your understanding, you may find that you may have focused too much on words rather than on words in context, which make meaning. You need to be careful and change this. As the saying goes, "words exist in context," because words out of context may mean nothing or too many different things.

- Taking notes during lectures/documentaries

Whether you are attending a health-related talk meant for the public in a university around your area (e.g. "Keeping Our Brains Young") or watching a documentary on TV (which discusses the topic in a more scientific way), take notes on what you listen. Imagine you need your notes to give a summary of the discussion/topic to someone who could not attend. As you will be focusing to take notes, you will notice that you will focus much more than if you were to just listen.

Additional activity on anticipation

Smokers at higher risk of losing their hearing, suggests study . . .
www.independent.co.uk/news/health/smoking-cigarettes-health-hearing-loss-study-japan-tokyo-tobacco-research-a8256856.html

1 Using the table below, make a list of ideas and terms (in English) which you believe will be used in talking about smoking

English terms about smokers and hearing	*How would I say this in my other language*

2 Then proceed to analyze the short text below and write your answers to the questions that apply to this text.

As well as annual health checks, some Japanese firms compensate staff who don't take smoke breaks

Smokers are not just putting themselves at risk of heart disease and cancer but may also be endangering their hearing, Japanese researchers have said.

A new study has found that current smokers were at a higher risk of hearing loss than nonsmokers – with that risk apparently increasing with each cigarette smoked. However, kicking the habit appears to reduce this risk again, the scientists said.

The authors said the findings provides "strong evidence" of a link, and called for new tobacco control measures to try and prevent or delay hearing loss.

The study, published in the journal *Nicotine and Tobacco Research*, tracked the lifestyle habits and health of more than 50,000 Japanese workers.

Using data drawn from records of annual health checks, which include a hearing test, the team looked at how workers' ability to detect both high and low pitch (frequency) sounds changed.

The results show smokers were 60 percent more likely to develop high-frequency hearing loss, compared to nonsmokers, and 20 percent more likely to lose some ability to hear lower frequency sounds.

One in ten workers developed some form of hearing loss over the eight-year study, and the more cigarettes a worker smoked each day the higher their risk of developing hearing loss, the study found.

"These results suggest that smoking may be a causal factor for hearing loss, although further research would be required to confirm this," the authors write.

Extratextual factors		*Write your answer here*
Who	Author of the text	
What for	Sender's intention	
To whom	Recipient/addressee	
How	Medium or channel	
Where	Place	
When	Time (text is written or read)	
Why	Motive	
Intratextual factors		
What	Subject matter, information presented in the text	
What not	Knowledge the author supposes that the reader has	
In what order	How is the text presented	
How	Words used, grammar, intonation	

3 Using the list of terms you have created in English and the information from the text itself, make a list of terms in your other language.

4 Using the list of terms in your target language and what you remember from the original text, make a speech in your other language.

5 Find information related to the topic at hand on the internet and complete your glossary of terms in English and the other language.

References

American Academy of Orthopaedic Surgeons (AAOS). (2013). "Patients Are Important Members of the Healthcare Team" This article is also available in Spanish: Los pacientes son miembros importantes del equipo de atención médica). Available at http://orthoinfo.aaos.org/topic.cfm?topic=A00271 (Last accessed May 1, 2017).

Angelelli, C. V. (2000). Interpreting as a Communicative Event: A Look through Hymes' Lenses. *Meta. Journal des Traducteurs*, *45*(4), 580–592.

______ (2001). *Deconstructing the invisible interpreter: A study of the interpersonal role of the interpreter in a cross- linguistic/cultural communicative event.* Ph.D. diss. Stanford University, Stanford, CA.

Angelelli, C. V., & Degueldre, C. (2002). Bridging the gap between language for general purposes and language for work: An intensive superior-level language/skill course for teachers, translators and interpreters: Chapter 4. In B. L. Leaver & B. Shekhtman (Eds.), *From advanced to distinguished: Developing professional-level language proficiency* (pp. 91–110). Cambridge, UK: Cambridge University Press.

Basnett, S. (1991). *Translation Studies*. London and New York: Routledge Taylor & Francis Group.

Burgess, H. (2013). Active listening. Available at www.beyondintractability.org/coreknowledge/active-listening (Last accessed March 3, 2018).

Council on Linkages between Academia and Public Health Practice. (2018). Definition of competency. Available at https://sph.uth.edu/content/uploads/2012/01/Competencies-and-Learning-Objectives.pdf (Last accessed May 7, 2018).

HealthRadio. (2018). Stress and mental illness. Available at www.healthradio.fm/audio/radio/151109_Jean-Paul-Gravel_Stress.mp3f (Last accessed April 13, 2018).

Matthews-King, A. (2018, March 15). Smokers at higher risk of losing their hearing, suggests study. Available at www.independent.co.uk/news/health/smoking-cigarettes-health-hearing-loss-study-japan-tokyo-tobacco-research-a8256856.html (Last accessed April 5, 2018).

Merriam Webster. (2018). Definition of competencies. Available at www.learnersdictionary.com/definition/competency (Last accessed March 9, 2019).

MSD Manuals. (2018). Which MSD manual is right for you? Available at www.msdmanuals.com/en-gb/ (Last accessed April 1, 2018).

Murphy, J. (1991, Spring). Oral communication in TESOL: Integrating speaking, listening, and pronunciation. *TESOL Quarterly*, *25*(1).

Nadin, M. (2018). Definition of anticipation. Available at www.anticipation.info/pages/definitions/index.html (Last accessed May 10, 2018).

Oxford English Dictionary. Definition of skill. Available at www.oed.com/view/Entry/180865?result=1&rskey=poxy5x& (Last accessed May 3, 2018).

Ranjan, P., Kumari, A., & Chakrawarty, A. (2015, March). How can doctors improve their communication skills? *Journal of Clinical and Diagnostic Research*, *9*(3), JE01–JE04. doi:10.7860/JCDR/2015/12072.5712. Epub 2015, March 1. Available at www.ncbi.nlm.nih.gov/pubmed/25954636 (Last accessed March 15, 2018).

Ray, L. (2017). Best exercise for morbidly obese people to lose weight. Available at www.livestrong.com/article/274887-best-exercise-for-morbidly-obese-people-to-lose-weight/ (Last accessed May 5, 2018).

Reiss, K. (1989). Text types, translation types and translation assessment. In A. Chesterman (Ed.), *Readings in translation theory* (pp. 105–115). Helsinky: Oy Finn Lectura.
Underwood, M. (1989). *Teaching listening*. London: Longman, 117 pp. ISBN 0582746191, 9780582746190.
US National Library of Medicine MedlinePlus. Available at https://medlineplus.gov/videosandcooltools.html (Last accessed April 13, 2018).
World Health Organization. (2017, December 4). Universal health coverage in Rwanda. Available at www.youtube.com/watch?v=GmQiA4J-XDw&feature=youtube (Last accessed February 12, 2018).

Further readings and resources

BBC for more information and a "fun" game on types of texts. Available at www.bbc.co.uk/skillswise/words/reading/typesoftext (Last accessed May 23, 2018).
Gavioli, L., & Baraldi, C. (2011). Interpreter-mediated interaction in healthcare and legal settings: Talk organization, context and the achievement of intercultural communication. *Interpreting*, *13*(2). pp. 205–233.
Gile, D. (2005). Teaching conference interpreting: A contribution. In M. Tennent (Ed.), *Training for the new millennium: Pedagogies for translation and interpreting* (pp. 127–151). John Benjamins Publishing.
Healthcare Interpretation Network (HIN). (2007). National standard guide for community interpreting services. Toronto, Canada. Copyright © 2007 Healthcare Interpretation Network. Available at www.healthcareinterpretationnetwork.ca and www.saludycultura.uji.es/archivos/HIN_National_Standard_Guide_for_CI_(Canada).pdf (Last accessed April 26, 2017).
Interpreter Training Resources. A resource for interpreters, students in interpreting and interpreter educators. Available at http://interpreters.free.fr/index.htm (Last accessed May 23, 2018).
Victoria State Government, Better Health Channel. (2018). Road and traffic safety. Available at www.betterhealth.vic.gov.au/health/HealthyLiving/road-and-traffic-safety-for-children (Last accessed February 12, 2018).

Further suggestions

Listen to or attend debates or political speeches on health matters. You may do any of the previous exercises with debates and political speeches and ask a few questions as to the intentions of the speakers, where they stand on certain issues, what are their goals, what are the connections between this event you are attending and what you know about the speakers or their health organizations/practices. This exercise will help you "read between the lines" and discover the implicit message behind what has been explicitly uttered. Political campaign speeches and debates on where a person stand on an issue of health services, language provision and so forth are good for this.

Attend (university) lectures with familiar and unfamiliar topics and analyze such material for discourse markers and rhetorical devices. Ask yourself what impact such devices have had on you as a listener. How can you use such devices in the future? Try to anticipate and predict future development in the segment. Usually structured speeches will be preferred to do this exercise, but finding your way through a convoluted speech is also beneficial.

In this chapter we have focused on some of the various competencies and skills involved on the reception side of interpreting (and communication): active listening, text analysis and anticipation. We have done some activities to develop those skills and stressed the importance of preparing for the encounter. While in this chapter and next we emphasize practice (guided and reflective practice, rather than practice and more practice), we have established clearly the link between research/theory and practice. This chapter and next exemplify that "learning without thought is labor lost; thought without learning is perilous" (Confucius).

6 Skills and competencies

Productive skills

With Christian Degueldre

GOALS

In this chapter we will:

- Familiarize ourselves with the skills and competencies involved in the production of a message in medical interpreting.
- Reflect further on the skills and competencies involved in interpreting in general and medical interpreting in particular.
- Focus on the productive skills (public speaking, paraphrasing, delivery).
- Discover the benefits of note-taking and sight translation in healthcare interpreting.

LEARNING OUTCOMES

By successfully completing this chapter, you will be able to:

- Understand the importance of self-monitoring.
- Differentiate between delivery and self-monitored delivery of information.
- Distinguish ways of processing shorter and longer segments of information.
- Use your memory effectively and improve your note-taking.
- Anticipate content and discover text structure in sight translation.
- Improve skills through exercises, practice, observation, analysis and reflection.

In Chapter 5 we examined the difference between skills and competencies. We have focused on the so-called receptive skills such as preparation, command of languages, active listening, discourse/text analysis and anticipation. In this chapter we focus on the productive skills such as public speaking and paraphrasing, as well as some other skills interpreters rely on to deliver a message: note-taking, memory, sight translation. We pay attention to skills specific to community/public-service interpreters and healthcare interpreters in particular, such as interpersonal skills. We conclude with some recommendations for further reading.

A. Productive skills

Skills associated with linguistic competence

Linguistic competence, as a concept, is associated with language proficiency. We discussed linguistic skills associated to listening in Chapter 5. On the productive side of interpreting, we focus on the ability to express oneself accurately in a culturally and socially appropriate way for the context in which we render the message. It means that interpreters must be able to express themselves in the ways of speaking of the parties for whom they work, using the correct technical and non-technical language, the appropriate register, body language and gestures, and use empathy appropriately to allow the parties to communicate effectively.

Public speaking skills

Interpreters' work implies performing for others. Interpreters speak/sign in front of others. Therefore, it is necessary to pay special attention to the skill of public speaking. Interpreters' work entails brokering the messages (utterances) of healthcare providers and patients to facilitate communication. Their professional performance is a major contributing factor to the success of cross-cultural communication. Interpreters work frequently between two parties (e.g. a healthcare provider and a patient). Sometimes they interpret for more than two. Examples of this may be when the patient is a child and the parents are present, or when the patient is accompanied by family members or friends, or when there is a provider and a nurse present or more than one specialist in the room or during a grand round.

Speaking in public requires paying special attention to our body language, our gaze, our gestures, our demeanor in general. Our bodies sometimes speak more eloquently than our voices. People notice when one is interested in what one is doing, when one shows genuine empathy, when one cares.

In addition to how one presents oneself, one will always perform better if one has prepared well. As we have discussed in Chapter 5, being prepared for an interpreting assignment is essential; it helps one to cope with problems and reduces the stress associated with public speaking.

Skills associated with interpreting competence

Paraphrasing for delivery

While interpreting during a doctor-patient encounter, many times interpreters face ways of speaking that are not their own and, most importantly, are not the patient's either. For example, the ways in which providers explore pain, request information on medical history and so forth, may differ from how patients from similar origin, socio-economic status or degrees of literacy do it (see Chapter 3). Based on their experiences, interpreters engage in paraphrasing and shift the register in which providers talk to make concepts more accessible to patients. Interpreters understand the meaning, they understand what the doctor is saying and they find a way to express it in the other language which, without altering the information, meets communicative needs. In these situations, interpreters give examples or explain that term/concept to the patient in different ways. Interpreters do this by keeping both parties informed of what they are doing.

Let us look at the following example. It comes from a database of authentic doctor-patient encounters (Angelelli 2018). In this case, the doctor recommends to a patient that she drinks only clear liquids. The interpreter identifies the term "clear liquid" as problematic, as one term that if she interprets literally the patient may not understand. She has several options. We can anticipate two typical ones: (1) either she provides an equivalent technical term in the other language (with the risk that the concept will not be understood by the patient); or (2) she brokers the understanding of the technical term by using an example. Let us see what the medical interpreter did in this situation:

Tape 28
105–211
"You can drink clear liquids only, well, when we say clear liquids, that means that when you put it [the drink] in a glass, you can see through without any problem" (Angelelli 2018).

The explanation that the interpreter decides to provide for the patient helps the patient understand better what the doctor was saying. The interpreter paraphrased. In this example, the interpreter made a conscious decision to explain to the patient what the term "clear liquids" mean. We know this fact because the interpreter was interviewed after the encounter so that she could talk about the challenges she faced and her performance. She stated that as soon as she heard "clear liquids" she realized that her rendering it in the same way, the same technical term in the same register, would not have been understood by the patient. Had the term "clear liquids" been understood by the patient, there would have been no need to provide any paraphrasing, but from previous experiences, the interpreter claimed that the patient would not know what "clear liquids" mean. So her goal was to make the term accessible to the patient.

As we see, paraphrasing is not a substitute for finding and using a correct term. Paraphrasing is to be used when needed. Learning to paraphrase makes interpreters more flexible as they have more options to work from using their languages. Let us look at some definitions of paraphrasing.

DEFINITIONS

The *Oxford English Dictionary* states that to paraphrase is to express the meaning of (something written or spoken) using different words, especially to achieve greater clarity (Oxford English Dictionary 2018).

Merriam-Webster's Dictionary defines paraphrasing as "a restatement of a text, passage, or work giving the meaning in another form," as in the example: the teacher asked the students to write a paraphrase of the poem.

Wikipedia defines paraphrasing as a restatement of the meaning of a text or passage using other words (Wikipedia 2018).

Another definition, provided by Purdue University (Purdue OWL 2018), states that one's paraphrasing is:

- One's own rendition of essential information and ideas expressed by someone else, presented in a new form.
- One legitimate way (when accompanied by accurate documentation) to borrow from a source (as we do when we write papers, for example).
- A more detailed restatement than a summary, which focuses concisely on a single main idea.
- It is not a summary. It is your own rendition of essential information and ideas expressed by someone else, presented in a new form.
- It does not contain words or phrases from the original (plagiarism).
- It includes all minor details from the original.
- The meaning of the writing being paraphrased is clearer to the reader than in the original text.
- It restates the thesis.
- It is usually as long as or longer than the original.

Generally paraphrasing is used to explain. Sometimes there is no need to explain because the original concept is relatively clear. Yet, for interpreters, paraphrasing is a useful exercise as it gives us the flexibility we need in our work.

We now look at some examples of paraphrasing which, although similar in content, are different in form.

Activity 1: paraphrasing

Look at the following three definitions of diabetes. What do they have in common? What can you learn from the comparison? Are they using a similar register? Are they of a similar or different level of difficulty?

Definition #1

Diabetes is a disease that occurs when your blood glucose, also called blood sugar, is too high. . . Insulin, a hormone made by the pancreas, helps glucose from food get into your cells to be used for energy (NIH 2018).

Definition #2

www.diabetes.org.uk/diabetes-the-basics

What is *diabetes*? *Diabetes* is a serious, lifelong condition where your blood glucose level is too high. There are two main types, Type 1 and Type 2 (Diabetes.UK 2018).

Definition #3

www.msdmanuals.com/en-gb/home/hormonal-and-metabolic-disorders/diabetes-mellitus-dm-and-disorders-of-blood-sugar-metabolism/diabetes-mellitus-dm

Diabetes mellitus is a disorder in which blood sugar (glucose) levels are abnormally high because the body does not produce enough insulin to meet its needs (Brutsaert 2018).

Comment: The three definitions contain fairly explicit ideas. They explain what diabetes is in a way that the public will understand. The goal of the message is to educate the public on diabetes. Those three definitions are very similar even though they have been produced separately and come from three different websites. Any one could be considered as a very good paraphrasing of the others.

We now will look at another example and do some practice:

Original sentence:

Glucose in the blood is produced by the liver from the foods you eat.

Options of paraphrasing may include (yours may be different):

- Our liver uses the food we eat to produce our blood glucose.
- The food that we eat is used by our liver to produce a substance which circulates in our blood: the glucose.

Activity 2: practice exercises in paraphrasing

Now is your turn. Follow these suggestions for individual work.

Remember: Let's do some practice now and be mindful of what we learned above: paraphrasing means using our own words. It is not sprinkling a few changes here and there. We change the whole sentence, even the sentence structure. We can do paraphrasing as an individual work or in pairs.

Individual work

Directions: Read the following passage once carefully, paying attention to the main idea and all the details it contains. Then put the text aside, and on a separate sheet, write down in your own words what you remember as if you were explaining the passage to a friend or colleague. You may also choose to speak into a digital recorder, instead of writing the answer down on a sheet of paper. Try to get a maximum of details and remember: it is not a summary!

In pairs: working with a partner

Directions:

1 Read the following passage once to your work partner, who should listen carefully, paying attention to the main ideas and all the details the message contains.
2 Ask your work partner to tell you in their own words what they remember as if they were explaining the passage to you for the first time. You listen carefully and compare their rendition to the original passage to check if there are differences or omissions. You may also choose to record the rendition into a digital recorder. This will allow you to listen to it later and compare to the original. Encourage your work partner to get a maximum of details and remember: one is not asked to provide a summary and should not use the same words as the original.

Paraphrasing a sentence/paragraph from a fact sheet educating the public on glucose:

Glucose in the blood gives you energy – the kind you need when you walk briskly, run for a bus, ride your bike, take an aerobics class and perform your day-to-day chores.

Now you paraphrase:

____

____

____

Possible suggestion:

When you exercise, or simply work around the house, when you run for a bus, use your bicycle or walk at a good pace, you spend energy – a lot of energy. That energy is given to you by the glucose in the blood.

Activity 3: choosing a text and paraphrase it individually or with a partner

Read the following passage once carefully, paying attention to the main idea and all the details it contains. Then, put the text aside (keep it close), and on a separate sheet, write down in your own words what you remember as if you were explaining the passage to a friend or colleague. You may choose to speak into a digital recorder, instead of writing the answer down. Try to get a maximum of details and, remember: it is not a summary!

Paragraph 1

Evidence that physical activity improves health is convincing, but we lack knowledge about how to increase physical activity in individuals and populations **(sentence 1)**. Taking part in sport may improve health, but sport is only taken up by a small proportion of the adult population, and mainly by the better educated **(sentence 2)**.

Now you try:

____

____

____

Suggestion 1

It is a well-known fact that good health is linked to physical activity. Less known, however, is how to increase physical activity in people and populations. One way is to do sport, but only a small portion of the adult population practices any kind of sport, and they are usually people with a better level of education.

Suggestion 2

Physical activity is a good way to stay healthy. The question that remains is how to increase the physical activity of people and populations, as we know that few adults practice any kind of sport and those adults are usually the best educated ones.

Comments

1 Notice that the number of sentences in both suggestions offered does not correspond to the original.
2 Notice also that both suggestions proposed are slightly shorter. This is unusual for a paraphrasing exercise. That is due to the fact that sentence #2 is basically a repetition with a small addition (one and a half hour) of sentence #1. There is no need to repeat it.

Activity 4: paraphrasing a longer text

Even low intensity exercise such as walking is associated with better health.

Evidence that physical activity improves health is convincing, but we lack knowledge about how to increase physical activity in individuals and populations. Taking part in sport may improve health, but sport is only taken up by a small proportion of the adult population, and mainly by the better educated.

> In this week's *BMJ*, a systematic review by Ogilvie and colleagues assesses the effect of interventions to improve walking on how much people walk, physical activity, fitness, disease risk factors and well-being. It found that interventions tailored to people's needs, which targeted the most sedentary or those motivated to change, can increase walking by up to 30–60 minutes each week.
>
> (Andersen 2007)

Now you try:

____

If you find this text is too long for a beginning exercise, you can split it in two or more parts.

Paragraph 2

In this week's *BMJ*, a systematic review by Ogilvie and colleagues assesses the effect of interventions to improve walking on how much people walk, physical activity, fitness, disease risk factors, and well-being. It found that interventions tailored to people's needs, which targeted the most sedentary or those motivated to change, can increase walking by up to 30–60 minutes each week.

Now you try:

Suggestion 1

In the current issue of our journal, Ogilvie and colleagues look at the impact of interventions on how to improve how much people walk. They also study other factors such as physical activity, fitness, risk factors for diseases and general well-being. Their conclusion was that with tailored interventions focusing on the most sedentary people and on the people who really are motivated to change, it is possible to increase the amount of walking time by up to 30–60 minutes a week.

Suggestion 2

A study by Ogilvie and colleagues published in BMJ this week focuses on interventions and their impact on how to improve the amount of walking people do per week. It shows that various factors such as physical activity, fitness, risks factors and well-being in general, when focusing on sedentary people and motivated people, can increase walking by up to 30–60 minutes per week.

Comments

1 Notice that both suggestions in this example use more words than the original.
2 Both use more, and shorter, sentences to express the ideas.
3 They also try to maintain the technical terms used in the original (i.e. physical activity, fitness, risks of diseases).

As discussed, paraphrasing is a valuable skill for interpreters. Paraphrasing a text makes us analyze its structure, its content and form. Understanding the structure, content and form helps us construct meaning. And without constructing meaning and understanding content and form, we cannot interpret.

By paraphrasing a text, we modify the form and, if needed, the structure of the message but not its content. We express the same ideas in a different way. We do not do this for the sake of doing it. We do this if it is necessary, as in the cases discussed above (to shift registers and make a concept more accessible, to give an example, to clarify). Learning to paraphrase is important as it is a relevant skill for healthcare interpreting (and for interpreting in general). We will revisit paraphrasing when we discuss sight translation.

Memory

In medical encounters, conversations between providers and patients vary in length. The variation occurs not only at the level of the whole conversation (may last from 10 or 15 minutes to 45 or more) but also at the level of each of the turns during the conversations. Turns between patients and providers vary in length from a few seconds to lengthier turns of several minutes. Interpreters must be able to keep a considerable amount of information in their short-term memory and reproduce it. This is the reason they need to take notes to support their memory. Managing our memory capacity and skill is important for the work of a successful interpreter.

The purpose of this segment is not to be exhaustive but to show the complexity of memory, the different types of memory and how these apply to interpreters. We hear often that "memory is like a muscle," even when research shows that the new learning occurs actually in the brain. Human memory is made up of multiple different systems that can all operate almost independently of each other (Squire 1996).

Figure 6.1 shows three types of memory: declarative, episodic and procedural. The declarative memory allows us to remember, for example, that insulin-dependent diabetic patients are Type 1 diabetic patients and that they need a regular uptake of insulin because their pancreas does not produce enough. The episodic memory tells us that last week during an encounter in which we interpreted, the patient, an 85-year-old woman, was telling the provider that she sometimes forgets to take her insulin. And the procedural memory allows that patient to remember how to prick her finger to test her blood glucose level.

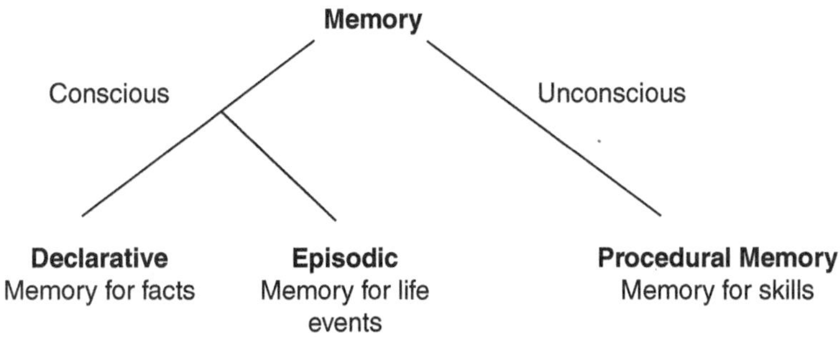

Figure 6.1 Muscle memory

Source: The Medium Corporation (2017); https://medium.com/oxford-university/the-amazing-phenomenon-of-muscle-memory-fb1cc4c4726.

Let us look now how interpreters use these different types of memories in their work. In his effort model (1995), Gile shows the prominence of the short-term memory (STM), and in his revised version of 2017 he introduces the concept of "working memory"; both are essential parts in the process of interpreting, which is an STM-centered activity. For Gile, the process of interpreting consists of "Encoding of Information from the Source Language + Storing Information + Retrieval of Information + Decoding Information into the Target Language" (Gile 1995, 2017).

The information is stored in STM in three different forms: (1) acoustic coding; (2) visual coding; and (3) semantic coding. All three forms combine to help the interpreter receive, understand and reproduce a message. Indeed, the interpreter must hear the message well (acoustic) and must grasp its meaning (semantic). To help the interpreter, there are many visual clues (the body language of the nurse, the hesitation on the patient's face, etc.). As we will see later in this chapter, the notes that interpreters take are also useful to assist in such visual coding of information, especially since their visual presentation reflects the structure of the ideas expressed by the provider-patient.

> The interpreter needs a good short-term memory to retain what he or she has just heard. . . and a good long-term memory to put the information into context. [Therefore] the ability to concentrate is a factor as is the ability to analyze and process what is heard.
>
> (Phelan 2001: 4–5)

Activity 1: practice for memory

When you listen[11] to the news every day, start listening as if you were to interpret each segment – that is, listen actively as an interpreter. In a 10-minute news broadcast, you might have heard information on five or six different topics. Write down on a sheet of paper one word that summarizes each topic. Then, without looking, put one finger on the page. The word that is closest to where your finger is pointing is the topic you will be working on. Take a minute to recall it, then present the information in the same manner you heard it first, trying to recall as many details as possible. Record the original in order to be able to compare both your version and the original. Note what you have been missing, the information you might have distorted and/or eventual addition(s) to the original message. When you listen to your recorded interpreting, pay attention not just to the content but also to the form (the pronunciation, the intonation, the register, the rhythm).

This exercise can be done with any type of information. It is better if the information is presented at a normal speed, is not too dense (i.e. does not contain too many details) and is not rehearsed. An extemporaneous discussion or a Q and A is better than a series of short 30-second segments, as the evening news sometimes presents.

Just like any skill, memory can be improved through exercises and practice.

Note-taking

We have just seen the importance of visual memory. We know that taking notes of dosage, prescriptions and appointments is a simple way not to overload the interpreter's memory. However, sometimes it is necessary to take more extensive notes in order to be able to remember a longer segment (two to four minutes or more) with all its details. This is possible thanks to a good note-taking system.

What does such a system look like? We first will draw from the following Guidelines for Note-Taking which were written not specifically for interpreters but for students in general, to draw some principles on note-taking:

> Concentrate on the lecture or on the reading material.
> Take notes consistently.
> Take notes selectively. Do NOT try to write down every word. Remember that the average lecturer speaks approximately 125–140 words per minute, and the average note-taker writes at a rate of about 25 words per minute.
> Translate ideas into your own words.
> Organize notes into some sort of logical form.
> Be brief. Write down only the major points and important information.
> Write legibly. Notes are useless if you cannot read them later!
> Don't be concerned with spelling and grammar.
> (Center for Teaching and Learning, Stanford University 2018)

For interpreters who received formal education in the field, the concept of note-taking is not new. It was first developed for conference interpreters. Indeed, the "basic seven principles" developed by Jean-François Rozan already in 1956 are present and re-visited in more contemporary works (e.g. Gillies 2017). Such a system allows an interpreter to take note of a relatively long presentation (10–15 minutes or more) without interrupting the speaker. Generally, in a patient-provider encounter the segments are relatively short. Healthcare interpreters usually do not need to interpret long segments, except maybe when they interpret an educational session (e.g. diabetes education). The notes are especially useful when interpreting descriptions of treatment, explanation of procedures and so forth. Developing a good note-taking system helps the interpreter as it reduces the demand placed on memory. The notes are simply a way to trigger the memory, forcing it to remember the concept(s) to which each note has been associated. An interpreter who takes notes not just of the numbers, dates and ingredients but of all the details of a speaker's utterance will see how the notes contribute to reducing the number of potential mistakes and improve the quality of the encounter.

The notes the interpreter takes make the skeleton structure of the speech more apparent. They are a visual representation of the ideas expressed by the speaker. They can be presented in a simple subject-verb-object (SVO) structure, as explained in the examples below.

Therefore the note-taking system allows the interpreter to write down more than the main ideas: it makes it possible to remember all the details and nuances of the message. Don't forget that the notes you take work in conjunction with your memory.

GENERAL PRINCIPLES OF NOTE-TAKING

If you look at the notes of different interpreters of the same message, you will notice that there are differences. But you will also see some basic principles. In Rozan's seminal work on note-taking, those are:

- *Noting the idea, not the word*: Interpreting translation (as well as translation) or any form of language mediation is about concepts and ideas, not about words. Once you understand a concept well, you create a mental image of that concept, which will later be uttered easily. If someone speak about a house, it is easier to draw a house than say "*maison, casa. . .*" Words need to be translated; concepts need to be expressed.
- *Use abbreviations* (and one can add "drawings"): Shorter forms of writing and more pictural ways to express an idea will give the interpreter more time and concentration to listen to the person who speaks. If someone talks about a white house, now you have the option of an abbreviation "WH," for example, or a drawing, whichever works best for you.
- *Links*: The different concepts of an utterance are usually (ideally) expressed in a structured way; you might benefit from noting the links between those ideas in a clear way, by writing the links in the margin of your page. The links may refer to cause, consequence, explanation or origin. Thanks to the link, the structure of the presentation is made more evident. Such links are "if," "thus," "if," "then," "but," "so," "because," "due to." The link can also take

the form of arrows to show in the case of an arrow pointing to the left, cause, and in the case of an arrow pointing to the right, consequence.

- *Negation*: Have a way to mark the difference between "there is no agreement" and "I disagree." When the doctor asks the patient if she has fever, listen carefully not to give the wrong answer and always write down the numbers you hear. It is easier to read a number you have written down than interpreting it in your head.
- *Emphasis*: Have a way to show the difference between "feeling just a little under the weather" or "feeling terribly sick," or between "having some pain" and "dying from pain." One way to mark those differences is to underline the concept (of pain) with one, two or three lines as the pain increases and one, two or three dotted lines as the intensity of the pain decreases.
- *Verticality*: Take your notes one idea on top of the next idea. This will allow for a more visual (structured) presentation of the speech.
- *Shift*: From left to right (and on the diagonal), try to jot down a representation of each idea presented following a simple "grammatical" structure of SVO (subject + verb + object).

Interpreters using Rozan's note-taking system have also found useful to add some more suggestions: (1) draw a line to separate two different ideas and two lines when the presentation from speaker A has finished; (2) when you have already taken note of an idea and if that same idea is repeated, use a line to connect the two points in your notes and bring the idea back instead of writing it a second time (only if you are on the same page of your notebook); (3) do not squeeze your notes on a single page – they would be more difficult to read back; (4) present your notes on the page in such a way that the concepts of parallel values appear at the same level (see our second page of notes below, where "couldn't walk, play football or go to school" are presented one below the other, at the same level of diagonality); (5) write down secondary/supporting ideas between brackets; (6) do not write too many things and rely also on your memory; and (7) adjust your note-taking system to your needs. If you interpret regularly for the pediatric unit at a children's hospital, you may develop different symbols than the one you will use if you interpret education sessions on diabetes at a local clinic.

Do not try to write down everything you hear. Note-taking is not another language replacing the target or source language.

Let us illustrate the principles described above on a real live story told by Mrs. Perez (a fictitious name) adapted for the requirements of this exercise.

Activity 1: note-taking. Visit to doctor for arthritis

In general, as part of the preparation for an encounter, the medical interpreter tries to get as much information as possible to help prepare. It is useful to get the name of the patient and the doctor or the name of the condition for which the patient is consulting. On that basis, the interpreter can read more about the condition on the internet or by other means in order to have a grasp of the condition and become familiar with some terms associated with it. The medical interpreter would write these on a separate sheet, with the abbreviation they plan to use in the notes and possibly the translation in the target language. Unfortunately, in this case, as this is a first visit, the clinical staff was not able to tell you anything. As an interpreter, you have been asked to come to Dr. Pope's office. You do not know what the purpose of the visit is.

When you get to the clinic, you are told that you are going to interpret for Mrs. Perez who has decided to come and see Dr. Pope because her daughter, Jimena, has been experiencing some pain. For the sake of this exercise, we will use the English version of what she reported to the doctor in Spanish. We take this conversation as Mrs. Perez starts explaining what she has noticed and why she is concerned.

Please look at our notes and read the comments that follow to see how the note-taking system for interpreters works. Remember it is a very individual system and it is based on each interpreter's memory.

Mrs. Perez: I came to see you because I am very concerned and I do not know what to do. A few weeks ago, I noticed that Jimena would wake up in the morning or first thing after a nap limping a little. . . not much. I asked her about it but she told me she was fine and did not feel any pain. I looked at her limbs and did not see anything abnormal. . . no swelling. However she seemed stiff. . . you know the way she would walk like having a stiff limb. I have not seen anything like this and do not remember anybody in my family or in my husband's family having anything like that. A few days ago, things got worse. Very often she could not walk, play as she liked to and even get out of bed. We thought she was stressed from things at school. But she started having some fever so I came to see you. We are very nervous because a girl of 13 shouldn't be in such a pain. Do you now know what she has?

Here is a suggestion for notes to help you interpret this message (Figure 6.2). As you take your own notes, pay attention to the form as well as the content of the message.

Comments on notes: On the top of the first page of the notes, it is a good idea to number the pages and to indicate into which language that segment needs to be interpreted into. Note that each "idea" or segment is separated from the next one by an horizontal line. This way ideas do not get mixed up during the delivery of the message. The presentation of an idea on the page is in diagonal following a "VOC" representation. Note that few words are used. This facilitates

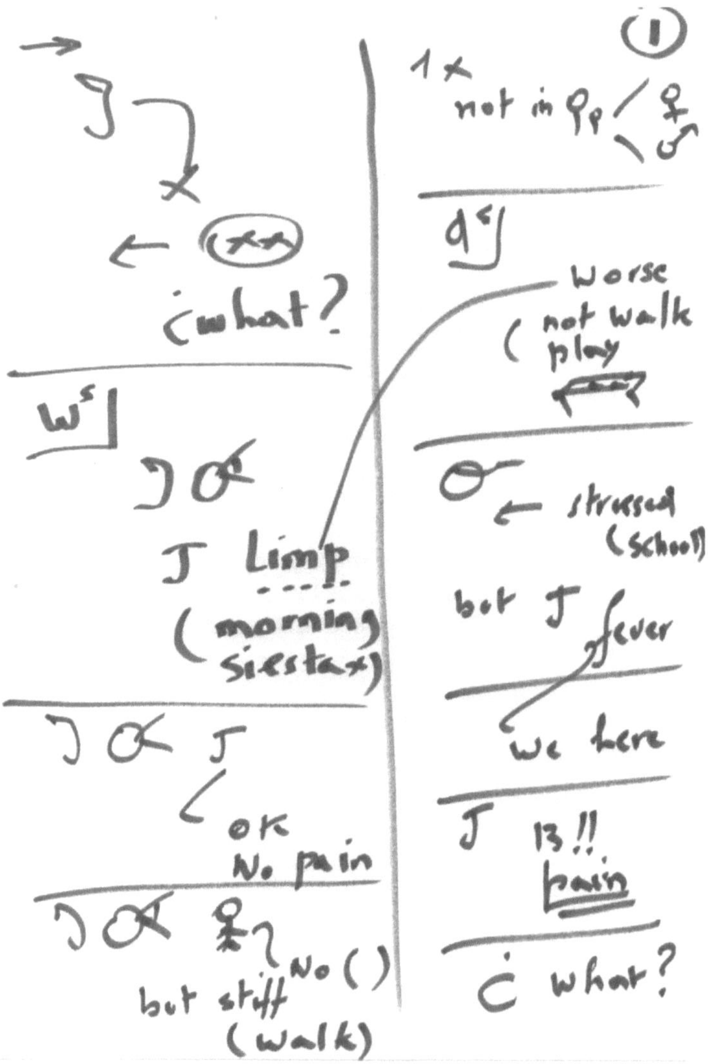

Figure 6.2 Note-taking 1

the "interpreting" phase as there is little "translating" involved. Some space is left on the left margin to indicate links between ideas (in this case, only one link: "but"). Let us examine the notes segment by segment. The left column below is an attempt to reproduce the notes; the right column explains what each annotation/symbol/abbreviation means. Do not forget that you do not need to take note of everything. You also rely very much on your memory when doing this exercise.

Segment 1:	*Meaning*
I	Mrs. Perez
arrow to the x linking I and x	Indicates movement
X	Place where you are now
. .	to express list of similar elements
arrow to the left	This arrow can mean movement or cause. It is cause in this example
Underlined face with two big eyes	The big eyes show concern, preoccupation. They are underlined to show the gravity of the concern
what?	Marks a question: what to do?

Segment 2:	*Meaning*
W	Abbreviation for week (time references can be only first letter. . . d = day; m = month; y = year)
s on top of w	Indicates plural
Symbol around w	Indicates time line. Vertical bar is for present. If it comes at the end of a horizontal line it means the element (w) is in the past. . . = weeks ago
I + face with an eye	I see (remember it is in the past) > I saw. .
J	Jimena (you decide what you use to represent the daughter. . . simple J initial is useful as her name may come more than once)
Limp underlined once in dots	Limp is left in English because there is no symbol that comes to mind to represent that idea
Underlined once in dots	The more underlines in dots decreases the importance of the symbol/word that is underlined. Only once in this case means that the limping was not significant/little.
Morning and *siesta* are in between brackets	Minor information is put in between brackets
X after *siesta*	x is a place taker. . showing in this case that it is right after *siesta*.

Segment 3:	*Meaning*
I face with a mouth + J	I told J (remember we are still in the past but there is no need to indicate it on the symbol)
Line from J going to the next part	Indicates that it is now J who speaks
OK No pain	J answered that she was fine and had no pain. The two elements are presented vertically one below the other to show similar levels.

Segment 4:	*Meaning*
I + face with an eye + drawing of little man	Indicates that Mrs. Perez is now looking at the legs of J
No ()	() represents an inflated leg
But	Put a little to the left to indicate opposition to previous idea
Stiff underlined once in dotted line	Indicates that the leg was a little stiff
(walk)	Minor idea in bracket

(*Continued*)

(Continued)

Segment 5:	*Meaning*
1x	Indicates the first time (such a thing was seen)
Not in big man accompanied by little person	Indicates family
Symbol for woman and men	Indicates the two families, of Mrs. Perez and her husband's. . .
Segment 6:	*Meaning*
D	Abbreviation for day (time references are only first letter. . . d = day; m = month; y = year)
s on top of d	Indicates plural
Symbol around d	Indicates time line. Vertical bar is for present. If it comes at the end of a horizontal line it means the element (w) is in the past. . . = days ago.
Line coming from segment 2 + worse	Indicates we are talking again about J and she has gotten worse
() with three elements placed as a vertical list	Minor elements in between brackets. . . not is not repeated as it applies to all three activities J is not able to perform any more
Segment 7:	*Meaning*
Head with a line coming out of it	I thought
Arrow to the left	Indicates causality
Stressed	Reason for the problem
(school)	Minor information in between brackets
But	Put a little to the left to indicate opposition to previous idea
J + fever	New elements: Jimena has a fever
Segment 8:	*Meaning*
line coming from fever	Fever is now the subject of the new idea; it is the cause of "we here"
Segment 9:	*Meaning*
J is 13	Indicate a fact
!!	Indicates exclamation, surprise
Pain is underlined twice	Indicates the severity of the pain
Segment 10:	*Meaning*
what?	Indicates a question: what to do? Being addressed now to the physician

Let us continue with the same story and listen to the response from the healthcare provider, Dr. Pope (a fictitious name).

> Dr. Pope: I have looked at all the symptoms and the tests we conducted. Jimena suffers from a condition which is not very rare but at the same time is serious. We do not know obviously how it is going to evolve because every

child is different. She suffers from a form of arthritis. In the United States about 300,000 children have some form of arthritis. It usually begins between the ages of 8 and 15. We need to conduct more tests and follow Jimena closely. We believe that Jimena suffers from what is called "juvenile idiopathic arthritis." It is the most common type of arthritis in children. *Idiopathic* means "of unknown origin." Be reassured: this disease is not contagious. We know it is more common in girls. It is just that we are uncertain what causes this disease. There is no evidence that foods or lack of vitamins play a role in developing the disease. Current research indicates that there is a genetic predisposition. We will follow how Jimena is evolving as we want to reduce the risks of serious complications such as eye or growth problems. . .

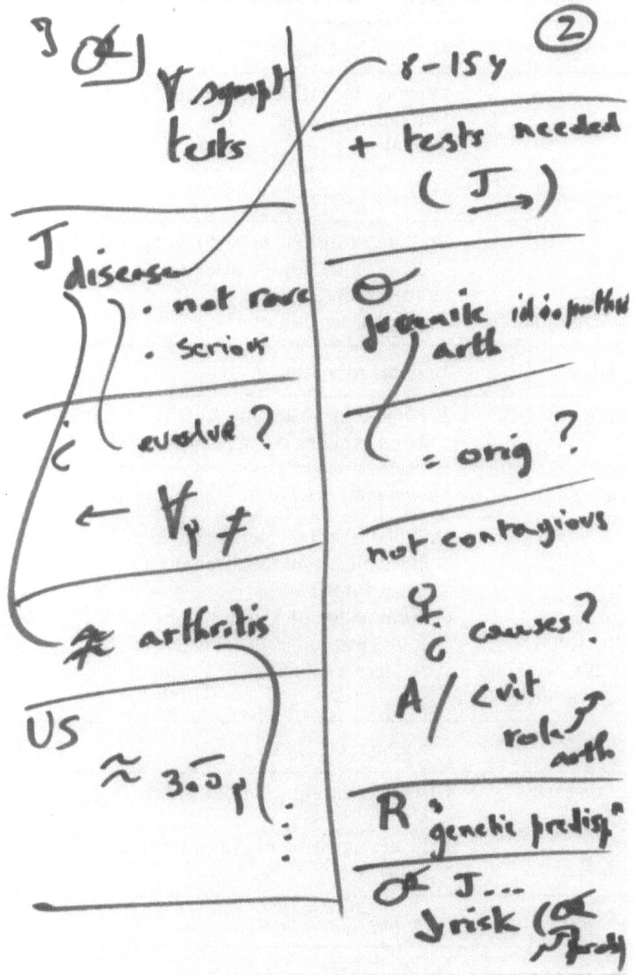

Figure 6.3 Note-taking 2

Take your notes and look at our suggestion in Figure 6.3. In note-taking, there is no right or wrong system. The only test of a good note-taking system (notice we limit the discussion to the ability to take notes) is if your notes are brief, clear and relevant so that you support your memory and are able to read them back in the foreign language.

Let us examine segment by segment the notes offered here above. You will notice the visual presentation on the sheet. It is airy; all ideas are separated by a line. It is simple.

Comments on notes above:

Segment 1: symbols	*Meaning represented*
I Face with an eye T sympt tests	Dr. Pope Looked at. . . Indicates the examination performed All symbols and tests are placed vertically as in a list to show equal level
Segment 2: symbols	*Meaning represented*
J Not rare serious	Jimena is the reference, the subject of the disease Two qualifying put vertically as in a list to show equal level
Segment 3: symbols	*Meaning represented*
evol? Arrow to the left T little person sign of not =	Dr. Pope is still the person talking, making a comment on the evolution of the disease Indicates causality All people are different
Segment 4: symbols	*Meaning represented*
Line + arthritis	The line brings back the "disease" element from segment 2 and explains it is a form of arthritis
Segment 5: symbols	*Meaning represented*
US Ondulated = sign 300 with bar on top + drawing of person Dotted vertical line with line bringing back "arthritis"	Dr. Pope is still the person talking, making a comment on the evolution of the disease Means "around" One bar on top of a figure multiplies it by 1,000 [line is equivalent to 000] so 2 bars would be 1,000,000 Introduces the concept of list/multiple types of arthritis
Segment 6: symbols	*Meaning represented*
Line bringing "disease" from segment 2 8–15 y	Disease is the subject of this idea Indicates age bracket of people affected by this form of arthritis
Segment 7: symbols	*Meaning represented*
+ tests needed J with arrow in brackets	No symbols here but words Indicates the need to follow J

Segment 8: symbols	*Meaning represented*
Head with line coming out of it	Expression of thought
Juvenile idiopathic arthritis	Write down the full name as this is a technical term

Segment 9: symbols	*Meaning represented*
Line from segment 8	Brings back the technical name of the disease
= orig?	Gives the meaning of idiopathic

Segment 10: symbols	*Meaning represented*
Not contagious	First element of a list
Symbol for female	Affects more girls
Causes is underlined in dots with interrogation marks	Question about the causes
A	Symbol for food
< vit	Less vitamins
Role + broken line going up	Role about the evolution of the disease

Segment 11: symbols	*Meaning represented*
R	Means research, as in R&D
“	Indicates talk/mention
Genetic predisp n	N on top of a word indicates it ends in -ion

Segment 12: symbols	*Meaning represented*
Head with eye	We will see
J. . .	Evolution of J
Arrow pointing down + risk	To reduce the risk
Up broken arrow + probl	Growth problems

Comments on the notes above: In this segment, we notice once again the verticality of the concepts which are at the same level. We also have lines in order to bring one unit from another segment on the page; different ideas are separated by a straight line.

We may take fewer notes on topics which are more familiar to us. However, regardless of how well we know a topic, we should take notes anyway, as (1) it is not our knowledge of the topic but rather what the speaker/signer states that makes the message; and (2) we do not know when the speaker will stop speaking and allow for the rendering.

Self-monitoring/assessing

Interpreting involves constant assessment of what we are doing. Being able to monitor our own production (after all, our renditions are the only things that count!) allows us to have better control over our production and the overall quality of our work. One way to improve our interpreting through self-monitoring is to record our own renditions as we practice; listen to each rendition and compare them to the original utterances. We may notice that our voice is dull, the message is presented in a convoluted way, it is choppy, unclear, the register is not appropriate, or we may have too unnecessary omissions in relation to the original. Such an exercise makes the interpreters more aware of how their work sounds.

Sight translation/sight interpreting

Sight translation consists of reading a text in one language and rendering it orally in another. It is a good pedagogical exercise that turns out to be very valuable for both translators and interpreters. It is considered an integral part of the recruitment process, together with consecutive and simultaneous interpreting, by international organizations (NATO Staff Interpreters 2002). In healthcare interpreting, you may use sight translation, for example, to give an oral version of a consent form before a surgery is performed, to sight translate some educational leaflets in diabetes educational sessions and so forth. If a diabetic nurse teaching a course on diabetes sticks to the text she has prepared and has shared with the interpreter in advance, the interpreter has the advantage of having it as a support text. They have some time to read it, prepare the terminology and understand the concepts.

Being able to use a text to do a quick sight translation is an advantage. We do not have to pay special attention to the figures as we have them in front of us; we may have written the translation of some difficult parts of the message to read our translation where the speaker gets to that point of the presentation.

On the other hand, having the written text can be a hindrance if we focus on it and lose track of the person speaking (the diabetic nurse, in our example). Listening to the speaker and at the same time following the text of the presentation and interpreting/sight translating it is multitasking. Interpreting is by definition multitasking, which demands a high level of concentration. If for some reason, the interpreter focuses on the text they are sight translating and does not listen to the speaker, there is a risk of getting behind the speaker and eventually having to sacrifice a sentence from time to time to catch up. Important information may be left out this way. Or, if focusing on the reading more than the listening, the interpreter may not realize that the speaker for one reason or another has modified the presentation to omit some parts or add to the text. All of these result in less quality interpreting As always, the interpreter is responsible for listening/following the speaker/signing because speakers/signers are the primary source of input for interpreters. A text for sight translation takes the part of a speaker, but if a nurse is explaining a brochure and reads aloud intersecting her comments, our attention is on the nurse's words. When she reads aloud we follow the reading, but we constantly check.

Another advantage of sight translation is that it can be used in lieu of a full written translation which might take much more time; a sight translation allows the interpreter to give a semi-polished version of the original text. The person who asks the interpreter to sight translate a text may not be interested in a full translation of the whole document but might be interested only in one segment or simply in understanding the gist of the message.

By learning how to do sight translation/interpreting we learn to anticipate the information ahead. We also learn how to analyze the message under pressure.

We verify our understanding of the main meaning and all the nuances of the message. We learn to multitask by sharing/dividing our attention between the text that we read and the oral delivery of it. We learn to make decisions while processing the original text and delivering its sight translation/interpreting version. When we sight translate/interpret a text, we need to make decisions in real time. This is an important skill to master. We may not always find an equivalent term in our target language and we need to provide a solution. Just like in simultaneous interpreting, we cannot stop the speaker. We have to use another way of expressing what we understood. We may not have a term but we may find a solution by using a synonym, a more generic term, or by paraphrasing. Sight translation/interpreting teaches us flexibility in our ability to render meaning in different ways. We gain mental agility.

HOW TO SIGHT TRANSLATE/INTERPRET A TEXT?

The first thing to do when you receive a text is to read it carefully – read it for the content and terminology. By doing this, we analyze the text, spotting the difficult parts that will require more attention. We may underline some key words that will trigger our memory from the first reading and will be useful when we sight translate the text. It is expected that our sight translation/interpreting rendition be smooth, without long interruptions, hesitations and/or backtracking. We should be flexible enough to recognize a difficulty in the text and find quick ways to go around it. And remember, sight translation/interpreting is not only about words!

Activity 1: sight translation

We will again use the topic of diabetes. There is virtue in repetition, because by now we either have familiarized ourselves with this health condition or we may want to read more about it in both source and target languages before we begin.

Instructions: We will split this exercise in four phases. Read all the instructions before beginning:

1 Using the link provided below, we will listen to the recording. As we listen, we pay attention to content and terminology. We may write down some terms we want to remember. As we listen, we analyze the message in order to understand it. After we finish listening, look at the terms you have written down and think of an equivalent in your target language.
2 This recording is accompanied by its transcription. Take the written text and sight translate it; try to maintain a regular rhythm; do not deviate from the meaning. Record yourself as you do this exercise.
3 Listen to the video and interpret it simultaneously. Record yourself.

4 Listen critically to both recordings you produced in numbers 2 and 3. Evaluate for meaning, speed, hesitation, tone, pronunciation, unnecessary additions and omissions of key or relevant information.

Here is the link: www.diabetes.org.uk/diabetes-the-basics

What is diabetes?

Diabetes is a serious, lifelong condition where your blood glucose level is too high. There are two main types, Type 1 and Type 2. They're different conditions, but they're both serious. There are some other rarer types of diabetes, too.

What causes diabetes?

What all types of diabetes have in common is that they cause people to have too much glucose (sugar) in their blood. But we all need some glucose. It's what gives us our energy. We get glucose when our bodies break down the carbohydrates that we eat or drink. And that glucose is released into our blood.

We also need a hormone called insulin. It's made by our pancreas, and it's insulin that allows the glucose in our blood to enter our cells and fuel our bodies.

If you don't have diabetes, your pancreas senses when glucose has entered your bloodstream and releases the right amount of insulin, so the glucose can get into your cells. But if you have diabetes, this system doesn't work.

Type 1 and Type 2

When you've got Type 1 diabetes, you can't make any insulin at all. If you've got Type 2 diabetes, it's a bit different. The insulin you make either can't work effectively, or you can't produce enough of it.

In both types of diabetes, because glucose can't get into your cells, it begins to build up in your blood. And too much glucose in your blood causes a lot of different problems.

To begin with it leads to diabetes symptoms, like having to urinate a lot, being incredibly thirsty, and feeling very tired. You may also lose weight, get infections like thrush or suffer from slow-healing wounds.

Complications

Over a long period of time, high glucose levels in your blood can seriously damage your heart, your eyes, your feet and your kidneys. These are known as the complications of diabetes.

But with the right treatment and care, people can live a healthy life. And there's much less risk that someone will experience these complications.

Get more information on living with diabetes.

Skills associated with cultural competence

Ability to navigate the cultural gap

The healthcare interpreter (as well as the cultural mediator) has to negotiate not just social and linguistic gaps but also cultural differences between healthcare providers and patients. As providers and patients may not be familiar with the social and cultural realities of each other, they may need help to bridge their beliefs and enable communication. Being able to understand the nuances of each culture, beyond cultural stereotypes, and communicate appropriately across the cultures is a skill required in professional healthcare interpreting.

As we discussed previously in Chapter 3, cultural differences and cultural competence are not limited to culture as associated with a language or place of origin of a person. We consider also the culture of healthcare providers as evidenced by their ways of speaking or as constrained by their duties and responsibilities; or the culture of patients, of lay people, whose life and decisions are based on other set of principles and beliefs than the providers' duties and responsibilities. The following situation is an authentic example of cultural clashing collected during fieldwork (Angelelli 2004). It illustrates cultural clashes and cultural competence gaps which occur in multicultural healthcare environments (Angelelli and Geist-Martin 2005).

It is an encounter between a genetic nurse and a pregnant woman, Ramira, who comes to the visit in her second month of pregnancy. She is over 30 years old. The nurse needs to explain to her that she has the option of doing a genetic test, an amniocentesis, to find out if the baby is healthy. During the explanation of the procedure, Ramira interrupts the nurse to indicate her concern about this test. The interpreter interprets this. The nurse explains to the patient that the amniocentesis is an option that patients have. It is not a required test. She also explains to the patient that healthcare providers need to present patients with their options. As the nurse continues to explain, she refers to a diagram that shows the places where the needle can be inserted. The nurse notices that the patient is expressing disagreement shaking her head "no." At that point the nurse emphasizes that the patient has a choice. She just needs to explain the test. The encounter has several interruptions to clarify issues, as misunderstandings occur in spite of the nurse trying to do what she is required to do, the patient listening, expressing her concern and attempting to do what she needs to do (avoid herself the stressful situation she was perceiving), and the interpreter interpreting the exchanges.

The nurse was frustrated as she was not trying to impose the test on Ramira; she needed to explain this option to her and to have her sign a form stating that she, the patient, was explained the procedure (regardless of her decision to accept or refuse the test). The patient did not want to listen to any more information about the tests because she had already had two miscarriages and she was determined to have the baby no matter what, provided the pregnancy would continue its course. The patient explained to the interpreter, who also interpreted for the provider, that there was no point in inserting a needle and posing any risk to the pregnancy to find out the information as she would not terminate the pregnancy even if the results were positive. After numerous attempts to continue (on the part of the nurse) and interrupt (on the part of Ramira) the session, it finally ended with the form signed. This was a powerful example of cultural communities clashing in front of the interpreter, as patient and nurse may not share expectation, beliefs and practices.

Interpersonal skills

In addition to all the linguistic, analytical and interpreting skills discussed, healthcare interpreters should exhibit good interpersonal skills. A healthcare interpreter relates with people all the time. The healthcare interpreter (just like the community or the court interpreter) is a participant in the interaction (be it face-to-face or on a screen) all the time. Having good interpersonal skills, beyond being polite, respectful and exercising good judgment, is an important factor in order to establish and maintain successful communication between all parties involved.

> A good interpreter is more than just a skilled linguist – he or she is someone who is willing and able to be a good, compassionate listener. Interpreting situations can be intimidating for non-native speakers, and an interpreter should try to make the experience as comfortable as possible. Second in importance to outstanding language skills is the ability to connect with a wide range of people.
>
> (Child 2017)

Building a good rapport with both the provider and the patient helps create a positive environment. For the provider as well as for the interpreter, being able to show empathy when needed without departing from the recommended ethics is a contributing factor to the success of the interpreter-mediated medical encounter. From a provider's perspective, empathy is described in the following way:

> you place yourself in your patient's situation and respond based on either similar personal experiences or through vicarious understanding. When you express empathy, it allows your patient to feel as though you understand his or her unique experience and that you are applying your expertise to the patient as an individual.
>
> (Srivastava 2014)

Skills associated with research competence

In contrast to translation, where the translator can stop the work to do research on the topic at hand, the interpreter needs to have completed the research before the actual assignment starts. Preparing for an assignment, understanding the concepts that will be discussed, becoming familiar with the different ways of speaking about them, identifying the appropriate terminology and knowing the ins and outs of the healthcare organization need to be done before the interpreting actually starts.

Healthcare interpreters should make appropriate use of the internet (differentiating between reliable and unreliable sources), the various terminology banks, the available databases, the relevant software and apps and all physical and virtual resources available to learn more about the topic they are going to interpret. Once the assignment starts, it is too late to do research. It is time to apply the research one has done.

As discussed in the previous chapters, in addition to using reliable available ones, we should build our own database of terms by preparing glossaries in our working languages. These can be in the form of Word files or Excel files, or any other form. They are personalized and may not be helpful to others, because they are the tools one designs to help oneself. They may be organized at different levels (e.g. by areas, by ailments, procedures, symptoms, or by need of the interpreter and, in general, in alphabetical order within each category). It is important that glossaries be easy to access and navigate, so that it is quick and easy to find a term.

Your research is not just about the terms; you need to understand the concepts. As an example, the term "empowerment" is not just difficult to translate but it is a concept that is not easy to grasp. Read about it to make sure you understand everything it covers and use the versions in other languages, when available and from a reputable source, to build up a glossary (Calvès 2009; Fischer & Amalia 2005; Narayan 2002). Keep track of useful, informative websites and make a note of what you like about them. Are they offering information in more than one language? Are they from a reliable source? In an open environment, everyone can upload information on the internet. And, once again, make sure that you do not waste your precious time in reading unreliable sources.

Skills associated with technical competence

Healthcare interpreters may work face-to-face or remotely. Working face-to-face is generally done in short consecutive (dialogue interpreting, as we discussed in Chapter 3), but from time to time it may require simultaneous done with portable equipment (e.g. a grand round with foreign experts who do not speak the societal language, a mixed marriage/family where one of the family members may speak a different language than the others). Familiarize yourself with the use of portable interpreting equipment (get your own if you can, or have your organization acquire one). Portable equipment allows the interpreter to work in simultaneous mode. This saves a lot of interpreting time. It is also a practical way to interpret for more than a couple of people when whispering/*chuchotage* is not possible.

When interpreters work remotely they may do so over the telephone (on site using speakerphones, wireless portable devices or dual-handle phones, etc.) or on videoconference calls. This requires the interpreter to know the technology on the one hand, and to know how to adjust to the input received on the other hand (audio and visual, audio only, etc.).

In addition, as discussed in Chapter 5 and earlier in this chapter, when we focused on various activities, we stressed the importance of getting into the routine of using a recording device (a digital recorder, or the recording device from the phone or the computer) to record exercises done as well as pictures of notes. Listening to one's performance is a powerful, humbling experience. It is one of the best ways to become aware of what you do well and not so well.

B. Research, observe and reflect

In this chapter, we have discussed some of the linguistic, interpreting, cultural, research and technical competencies that interpreters have and some of their associated skills. In this exercise, we bring together all the information we have learned about the skills interpreters acquire to perform professionally.

We will read part of a transcription segment of an authentic interpreted communicative event. This is an example of interpreting performed in real time. Now we have the possibility to analyze the performance, to put it under the microscope. The interpreter in real time could not do this. The idea is not to judge good or bad interpreting but to learn to analyze this interaction. Later we can do the same with ours.

We will focus on the skills the interpreter uses. We will list them and analyze them. In addition, we will ask ourselves the following questions: had I been the interpreter, would I have performed in the same way? Would I have done things differently? If so, how? And why? We will identify what we see as successful performances on the part of this interpreter. We will justify our comments by applying what we have learned (what skill was used, what result was obtained, etc.). To do this, we remember that interpreting is a situated practice and it is a form of communication. We do not focus on one term or one behavior as an indicator of success or failure. We focus on larger and smaller units, and we list them all. We focus on achieving the communicative goal, on the messages getting across, on strategies used to accomplish them; we focus on having the appropriate language level, in coordinating the turns of conversation, in register shifts, in adapting language to each party and so forth. We will also list the issues that caused problems.

This background information will help us contextualize the transcript. The interpreter, Marta (a middle-aged Mexican woman), works as a full time interpreter for the hospital, in the language services unit. She joins the interview remotely through the speakerphone. The patient is a young male. Marta interprets between him and the female doctor. The visit is to discuss the results of a recent ultrasound. The patient is concerned about the results as they reveal a problem in a testicle.

Tape 69 – Marta side A call 2 168–244

1 I Okay
2 D Okay, I just wanted to discuss what we see on the ultrasound.
3 I *Okay, buenos días Carlo* [*sic*], *eh, Jorge.*
Okay, good morning Carlo [*sic*], hmmm, Jorge
4 P *Buenos días.*
Good morning

5 I *¿Cómo ha estado? Yo le voy a ayudar a interpretar para Beth que está con usted, me llamo Marta. Ready*
How are you? I am going to help you with the interpreting for Beth who is with you now. My name is Marta. Ready.

6 D Okay, it's just that, the ultrasound did not show anything really to worry about at all.

7 I *Dice que el ultrasonido, verdad, no les está enseñando de lo que, por lo que se tengan que preocupar. Ellos no ven nada, verdad, por lo que haya que preocuparse*
She says that the ultrasound, well, is not showing anything, anything one should worry about. They do not see anything, right, for which you should be concerned.

8 D I was checking to see if there's was any kind of a big tumor, or ah, like an abscess or anything like this that would cause the pain and there really isn't anything.

9 I *Dice que ellos. . . vieron. . . estudiaron el ultrasonido querían ver si había algún tumor, algún absceso, o algo verdad que les diera un poquito de información pero no hay nada.*
She says that they saw. . . checked the ultrasound. . . she wanted to see if there was any tumor, any abscess, anything, right?, that would give them information, any indication. . . but there is nothing.

10 D Okay, so I think we were right, the infection may be in the epitomes on the tube alongside of his testicles.

11 I *Bueno, okay, dice que entonces ahora ellos están un poco más seguros verdad dice que el. . . el. . . la infección puede estar en el conducto señor que va al testículo.*
Well, okay, she says that now they are a little bit more certain, right. She says that the, the, the infection can be in the main tube that goes to the testicle.

12 D Okay, so he should finish up the antibiotics.

13 I *Por favor, usted debe continuar tomando su antibiótico.*
Please you must continue taking your antibiotics.

14 P (inaudible 185) *y cómo, ¿se me va a quitar o qué?*
(inaudible 185) and how, is it going to go away by itself. . . or. . . what?

15 I *Eh, no le entendí señor.*
Hey, I did not understand you sir.

16 P *¿En qué me puede afectar o, se me, se me puede quitar eso o cómo se sigue. . ?*
How can it affect me or, can I, can it be removed. . . or. . . what is next?

17 I *Okay, ¿quiere saber usted si se le va a aliviar o si le va afectar otra cosa?*
Okay, you want to know if you will be relieved or if it is going to affect anything else?

18 P *Sí.*
Yes.

19 I *Okay. Doctor, he wants to know if that problem will go away completely or if that's gonna* [*sic*] *affect him in another way?*

20 D No, it should not be affecting him sexually. If it doesn't keep getting infections.

21 I *Dice, para empezar, sexualmente esto no le debe afectar.*
She says, to begin with, sexually this should not affect him.

22 D The discomfort may never completely go away, it may with time.

23 I *Okay, dice que la molestia que siente ahí verdad quizá se le quite con el tiempo pero también existe la probabilidad que nunca se le quite completamente.*
Okay, she says that the discomfort you feel there may well disappear over time but there is also the likelihood that it will never go away completely.

24 D That's why I told him, if it starts to swell again he should change the Motrin, the anti-inflammation medicine.

25 I *Es por eso que ellos le recomendaron verdad, que si le mole* [*sic*], *si le sigue molestando, si continúa molestando, debe de tomar el, umm, el Motrin verdad, y el antinflamatorio.*
That's why they recommended you, right, that if this is bothe [*sic*], if it continues to bother him, if it continues to bother, you should take the, umm, the Motrin, right, and the anti-inflammatory.

26 P *Okay, pero, ¿esto no es nada malo o sea no me afecta en nada? ¿El dolor nunca se me va a quitar pero no me afecta en nada?*
Okay, but this is not something bad, I mean it is not affecting me at all? The pain is not going to go away but it does not affect me in another way, right?

27 I Emm, he's asking the same question, do you think that it's gonna [*sic*] affect him in another way?

28 D What does he mean in another way? I just explained it, so what does he mean?

29 I *Okay, ¿en qué otros aspectos señor piensa que le puede afectar porque ya le explicó ella?*
Okay Sir, in what other ways do you think it could affect you because she has already explained. . .

30 P *Por ejemplo cuando tenga hijos o algo.*
For example about having children or anything.

31 I *Ella le dijo que en la vida sexual no le va afectar, verdad.*
She told you that your sex life will not be affected, right.

32 P *Oh.*
Oh.

33 I Okay, yeah, like to have babies, just to procreate.

34 D Again, if anything he needs to prevent himself from getting reinfected and reinfected by using condoms.

35 I *Okay, dice que en qué forma usted va a protegerse verdad, usted se va a proteger usando condones para evitar infectarse de nuevo.*
Okay, she says how are you going to protect yourself, is. . . right. . . you're going to protect yourself by using condoms to avoid getting infected again.

36 P *Oh sí, yo sé.*
Oh, yes. I know.
37 I *Okay, es la forma que ella quiere que usted se cuide, que se proteja.*
Okay, this is the way she wants you to take care of yourself, to protect yourself.
38 P *No, ya sé, pero o sea por ejemplo, yo estoy por casarme o sea ¿qué me puede afectar eso o qué?*
No, I know, but that is, for example, I am about to get married, that is, can this affect me or what?
39 I *Eh, es lo mismo que ella le dijo. He's asking the same question, he's saying he's going to get married and he wants to know if that something can happen.*
Hey, she already told you this. He's asking the same question, he's saying he's going to get married and he wants to know if that something can happen.
40 D If that something could happen, I don't know what you mean.
41 I *¿En qué aspecto tiene miedo señor?*
What are you afraid of, sir?
42 P *En que la pueda contagiar o. .*
In that I can infect her or. . .
43 I Oh, okay, and he thinks (inaudible 213) and he's gonna [*sic*] transmit it to his future wife.
44 D If he does not use condoms when he's out messing around, yes, but as far as what he had I think we have taken care of it.
45 I *Dice que, em, si usted no se cuida cuando tenga el problema, sí la puede contagiar, por ahorita ellos están tratando de darle este tratamiento al problema pero usted es el que va a tener que poner de su parte en el futuro.*
She says that, emmm, if you do not take care of yourself when you have the problem, yes you could infect her, right now they are trying to give you this treatment for the problem you have but you are the one who will have to be careful in the future.
46 P Okay.
47 I *¿Okay? ¿Sí entendió verdad?*
Okay? You did understand, right?
48 P *Sí.*
Yes.
49 I Okay, yes he understood.
50 D Very important and until he gets into a relationship where he's with one woman only, he needs to use condoms, so he doesn't keep reinfecting himself.
51 I *Señor, es muy importante, muy importante que usted tenga relaciones sexuales solamente con una persona.*
Sir, it is very important, very important that you have sexual intercourse with only with one person.
52 P *Okay.*
Okay.

53 I *Y se proteja porque si no usted se va a seguir contagiando y puede contagiar a otra persona.*
And that you protect yourself because if you do not, you will continue to be infected and you can infect another person.
54 P *Okay.*
Okay.
55 I Okay.
56 D Okay? Alright, so, if it gets a little swollen again, the Motrin, becomes a chronic problem, bad, bad pain like he was having before he might one to get followed up but I think he's on the right track.
57 I *Dice que ella piensa verdad que usted ya está, ya lo llevan más a o menos por el camino que debe de ser, pero si usted necesita algo para el dolor o para desinflamar use el motrin por favor y también usted se va a dar los asientos de agua que ellos le indicaron. Si usted continúa con dolor fuerte de nuevo, por favor regrese pero ella no piensa que ya eso va a pasar.*
She says that she really thinks you are ok, that you more or less where you should be, but if you need something for the pain or to reduce inflammation use the motrin, please, and you will also take the water seats as they indicated. If you continue to have severe pain, please come back but she does not think that is going to happen.
58 P *No, no, no, de hecho no se me ha inflamado no mas (sic) a veces siento un poquito de molestias pero no tengo inflamación ni nada.*
No, no, no, in fact I have not had any more inflammation, not any more [*sic*] sometimes I feel a little bit of discomfort, but I do not have inflammation or anything.
59 I He said that he doesn't have any more swelling only a little bit bothered, uncon [*sic*], something uncomfortable. . .
60 D Okay, alright, he may wanna [*sic*] continue the Motrin for a little while then if it's, if it's that way, but I, but I think the antibiotics it's really pretty much helped to take care of the problem.
61 I *Por favor, dice que ella quiere que continue tomando por ahorita todavía el Motrin si usted todavía tiene poquita molestia.*
Please, she says she wants you to continue to take the Motrin for now if you still have a little of discomfort.
62 P *Okay.*
Okay.
63 I *Dice para tratar de ayudar con eso, a ver si se siente mejor y tómelo hasta que ya no le moleste.*
She says to try with Motrin and see if it helps you with this, see if you feel better and take it until it does not bother him anymore.
64 P *Okay.*
Okay.
65 D Don't worry.
66 I *Y por favor, no se preocupe.*
And please, do not worry.

67 D Okay.
68 I *No se preocupe mucho, ¿okay?*
Do not worry much, okay?
69 P *Okay.*
Okay.
70 I *Okay.*
Okay.
71 D Thank you.
72 I You have a good day doctor.
73 D You too.
74 I Okay, bye, bye.
75 P Bye, bye.
Duration: Approx 45 min

What can we observe in this interaction and in Marta's performance?

We discuss two examples, one at the micro and one at the macro level. The rest of the transcript can be used to answer the questions we posed at the beginning.

At the micro level, we note how some medical terms used by the nurse such as "epitomes" (turn 10) are simplified by using "*conducto*" (conduct/tube) or explained by the interpreter when she accompanies them with a more colloquial synonym as in "Ok, ok like having babies, to procreate" (turn 33).

The interpreter constantly monitors each party's understanding and what each one wants to achieve from the interaction. On turns 12 and 13, the nurse and the interpreter are talking about continuing antibiotics, but the patient has something else on his mind. He is concerned about the impact on his sexual life (made explicit in turn 14). This actually is the patient's main concern (as stated in a post-interview), while the nurse is focusing on the condition itself and its treatment.

On turn 38, the patient explains his concern because he is about to get married and asks the nurse if "something can happen." On turn 39, the interpreter takes upon herself to repeat that the nurse has already answered his question when she turns to the nurse saying "he is asking the same question." The nurse does not understand Jorge's concern. The interpreter intervenes and asks the patient why he is afraid.

The nurse repeats that he should use condoms, adding "when he's out messing around" (turn 44). This is something that the interpreter decides to leave out. This allusion comes back at turn 50 when he is told to limit his "relationship with one woman."

At the macro level, Marta's performance is a good example of showing empathy. She actively listens to both parties, she is sensitive to what each is saying (and not saying) to each other. She avoids any potential, unnecessary tension. She brings both the patient (concerned with the impact on his sex life, his ability to have children and the possibility of infecting his future wife) and the nurse who is concerned about the treatment, the result of the ultrasound, the use of anti-inflammatory Motrin and the protection with condoms. By the end of the consultation, the patient knows what to take and is told and reassured that he should not worry.

C. Journal writing

In Chapters 5 and 6, we have discussed different skills healthcare interpreters use. We have encouraged you as our reader to reflect on these skills, how you can use them, what they are for and how you can work on them. As you do that, we encourage you to keep a journal of your practice. You may be familiar with logs. We ask you to do this entry at two levels:

1 Write down what you do on a regular basis when you do exercises on active listening, when you paraphrase or sight translate a text, when you practice note-taking, memory and so forth (providing as many details as you can on the skill you practice, when you practice, with what materials, for how long, in what language direction, etc.).
2 We ask you to add to the logging of the activities a journal entry about your self-guided reflective practice. In addition to the basic information about your practice (point 1 above), we want you to include your analysis. This is different from judging what you do as a good or a bad performance. Analyzing your interpreting means asking questions and reflecting on the answers, understanding what you did, why you did it, what purpose it served, what issue it caused and so forth. By constantly reflecting on your practice, by becoming aware of what you do that enables you to perform better or what you do that causes you an issue, you will know the areas in which you need to focus more to achieve better results.

D. Further tasks

Sight translation: research and practice

This exercise is about practicing sight translation of medical materials and forms generally found in hospitals. We will do it in two parts:

Part 1: You will visit and observe a hospital or clinic nearby. You will approach the reception counter, introduce yourself and explain the purpose of your visit. You will take a look at the educational brochures they may have for patients and ask if you can have samples. You will also inquire about the documents which are routinely handled to patients to read and sign. You will ask if you could have samples or if you could be directed to the office that may allow you to get/download some of these documents. As you are in the clinic/hospital you will observe in which languages information is offered, if any one beyond he societal language, write down the languages. Make sure, if available, you get the materials in your language combination.

Part 2: You will select one topic among the ones you may have gathered (a presurgical consent form, a medical history questionnaire, etc.), research the documents, the content, the terms, the register and so forth. You will then proceed to practice sight translation and record yourself. You then will compare your rendition with the content and forms/documents you have gathered in the other language.

References

Andersen, L. B. (2007). Physical activity and health. *BMJ, 334*, 1173. Available at www.bmj.com/content/334/7605/1173 (Last accessed June 10, 2018).

Angelelli, C. V. (2018). Can ethnographic findings become corpus-studies data? A researcher's ethical, practical and scientific dilemmas. *The Interpreter's Newsletter*, (22): 1–15.

———. (2004). *Medical interpreting and cross-cultural communication*. London: Cambridge University Press.

———. (2001). *Deconstructing the Invisible Interpreter: A study of the interpersonal role of the interpreter in a cross- linguistic/cultural communicative event*. Ph.D. diss., Stanford University, Stanford, CA.

Angelelli, C. V., & Geist-Martin, P. (2005). Enhancing culturally competent health communication: Constructing understanding between providers and culturally diverse patients. In E. B. Ray (Ed.), *Health communication in practice: A case study approach: Chapter 22* (pp. 271–284). NJ: Lawrence Erlbaum Associates.

Brutsaert, E. F. (2018). Diabetes mellitus (DM). Available at www.msdmanuals.com/en-gb/home/hormonal-and-metabolic-disorders/diabetes-mellitus-dm-and-disorders-of-blood-sugar-metabolism/diabetes-mellitus-dm\ (Last accessed May 3, 2018).

Calvès, A.-E. (2009). Empowerment: The history of a key concept in contemporary development discourse ("Empowerment": généalogie d'un concept clé du discours contemporain sur le développement"). *Revue Tiers Monde, 200*(4), 735–749. Available at www.cairn.info/article.php?ID_ARTICLE=RTM_200_0735

Center for Teaching and Learning: Stanford University Guidelines for Note Taking. Available at https://web.stanford.edu/dept/CTL/Student/studyskills/taking_notes.pdf (Last accessed March 10, 2018).

Child, J. (2017). 5 Qualities every interpreter should have. Available at http://daily.unitedlanguagegroup.com/stories/editorials/5-qualities-every-interpreter-should-have (Last accessed March 3, 2018).

Diabetes.UK. What is Diabetes. Available at www.diabetes.org.uk/diabetes-the-basics (Last accessed May 3, 2018).

Fischer, P., & Amalia, E. (2005). Les chemins complexes de l'autonomie. *Nouvelles Questions Féministes 24*(2), 62–85.

Gile, D. (2017). The effort models and gravitational model: Clarifications and update 2017.02.16 version with updates on the social situatedness of the EMs and risk assessment. Available at www.cirinandgile.com/powerpoint/The-Effort-Models-and-Gravitational-Model-Clarifications-and-update.pdf (Last accessed May 15, 2018).

Gile, D. (1995). *Basic concepts and models for interpreter and translator training*. Amsterdam and Philadelphia: John Benjamins.

Gillies, A. (2017). *Note-taking for consecutive interpreting: A short course*, 2nd edition. London and New York: Routledge Taylor & Francis Group.

The Medium Corporation. (2017). Oxford university: The amazing phenomenon of muscle memory. Available at https://medium.com/oxford-university/the-amazing-phenomenon-of-muscle-memory-fb1cc4c4726 (Last accessed July 7, 2018).

Narayan, D. (2002). *Empowerment and poverty reduction: A source book*. Washington, DC: World Bank. [*Autonomisation et réduction de la pauvreté*. Washington, DC: World Bank, 2004].

NATO Staff Interpreters. (2002, July 2) Recruitment of interpreters at NATO. *aiic.net*. Available at http://aiic.net/p/291 (Last accessed May 3, 2018).

NIH-National Institute of Diabetes and Digestive and Kidney Diseases. What is Diabetes. Available at www.niddk.nih.gov/health-information/diabetes/overview/what-is-diabetes (Last accessed May 2, 2018).

Oxford English Dictionary. (2018). Available at https://en.oxforddictionaries.com/definition/paraphrase (Last accessed July 3, 2018).
Phelan, M. (2001). *The interpreter's resource*. Clevedon, Buffalo, Toronto, and Sydney: Multilingual Matters Ltd.
Purdue OWL. Definition of paraphrase. Available at https://owl.english.purdue.edu/owl/owlprint/619/ (Last accessed May 15, 2018).
Rozan, J.-F. (1956). *La prise de notes en interprétation consecutive/Note-taking in consecutive interpreting*. Geneva: Georg.
Squire, L. R., & Zola, S. M. (1996). Structure and function of declarative and non-declarative memory systems. *Proceedings of the National Academy of Sciences, 93*, 13515–13522.
Srivastava, S. B. (2014). The patient interview. In C. D. Lauster & S. B. Srivastava (Eds.), *Fundamental skills for patient care in pharmacy practice*. Burlington: Jones and Bartlett Learning. Available at http://samples.jbpub.com/9781449652722/9781449645106_ch01_001_036.pdf (Last accessed May 14, 2018).
Wikipedia. Definition of paraphrasing. Available at http://en.wikipedia.org/wiki/Paraphrase#Pedagogy (Last accessed May 15, 2018).

Further readings

Akbari, A. (2017). Needed skills and strategies to improve the efficiency of sight translation in classroom context. *Trans-Kom, 10*(1), 22–44.
Chmiel, A. (2010). How effective is teaching note-taking to trainee interpreters? *The Interpreter and Translator Trainer, 4*(2), 233–250.
Gillies, A. (2017). *Note-taking for consecutive interpreting: A short course*, 2nd edition. London and New York: Routledge Taylor & Francis Group.
Gorm Hansen, I., & Dragsted, B. (2009). Exploring translation and interpreting hybrids: The case of sight translation. *Meta, 54*(3), 588–604.
Heinz, M. (2010). Improving the public speaking dimension of interpretation skills through English support courses. *Interpreting and Translation Studies, 13*(2), 251–265.
Lambert, S. (2004). Shared attention during sight translation, sight interpretation and simultaneous interpreting. *Meta, 49*(2), 294–306.
Lee, J. E. (2012). What skills do student interpreters need to learn in sight translation training? *Meta, 57*(3), 694–714.
Lung, R. (1999). Note-taking skills and comprehension in consecutive interpretation. *Babel, 45*(4), 311–317.
MSD Manuals. Available at www.msdmanuals.com/en-gb/ (Last accessed April 3, 2018).
Nolan, J. (2005). Interpretation: Techniques and exercises. Clevedon and Buffalo: Multilingual Matters.
Orlando, M. (2014). Implementing digital pen technology in the consecutive interpreting classroom. In D. Andres & M. Behr (Eds.), *To know how to suggest. . . Approaches to teaching conference interpreting* (pp. 171–199). Berlin: Frank & Timme GmbH.
Skillswise. Available at www.bbc.co.uk/skillswise/topic/format-and-style/resources/e3 ©BBC Copyright (guidelines about types of texts).
Timarová, Š. (2008). Working memory and simultaneous interpreting. In P. Boulogne (Ed.), *Translation and its others*. Selected papers of the CETRA Research Seminar in Translation Studies 2007. Available at www.arts.kuleuven.be/cetra/papers/files/timarova.pdf

7 Understanding the role of healthcare interpreters

GOALS

In this chapter we will:

- Explore the evolution of interpreters' roles.
- Learn about the various conceptualizations of interpreters' roles.
- Explore how interpreters perceive their role.
- Reflect how other people see interpreters' role.

LEARNING OUTCOMES

By successfully completing this chapter, readers will be able to:

- Analyze the many roles interpreters play.
- Discover how metaphors are used to describe the interpreters' roles.
- Learn how the co-participants in the medical encounter perceive interpreters' roles.
- Learn about the importance of education in shaping interpreters' roles.

In this chapter, we discuss the role of healthcare interpreters. It is a topic that has attracted much attention in healthcare interpreting. The role interpreters play during an interpreted communicative event may have direct impact on the technical (medical) as well as personal information transmitted during the interactions (Angelelli 2004a: 78). Together with ethics, role may be one of the most provocative topics in the field. Like the role of the translator, the role of the interpreter has changed significantly across time. It has evolved as a result of empirical research. In healthcare settings, the role of the interpreter is dynamic and fluid. Like the practice of interpreting, it is contextually bound. In this chapter, we will explore the role of the healthcare interpreter from different perspectives. The exploration is grounded in a growing body of research that looks at role in all its dimensions and shows the metaphors used by interpreters themselves to refer to their practice. We will discuss how role is perceived by the interpreters themselves, by the other co-participants to the interpreted communicative event (patients, providers), by the professional associations and by the parties hiring the services of interpreters. We will explore the behaviors and consequences of the various roles medical interpreters can play. Institutional/personal expectations of the role will also be discussed.

A. Tracing different conceptualizations of role

As a result of empirical studies, the understanding of the role of the interpreter (and of the practice of interpreting) has evolved significantly over the last 20 years. In the 1970s, the interpreter was considered to be a transmitter of information into a different language. This conceptualization was in line with the conduit model of communication (Reddy 1979). According to this model, the role of the interpreter is similar to that of a language modem (modulator/demodulator) that changed languages. This conceptualization of the role of the interpreter is in alignment with one of the first theories of interpreting, *la Théorie du Sens* (Seleskovitch and Lederer 1984). This theory has been important in calling attention to a practice that until then had been unnoticed. It does contain, however, several underlying assumptions about communication, understanding and so forth, and the role that interpreters play. These assumptions have been challenged by empirical research. The following are some examples of these assumptions:

1 Communication is monolithic and linear.
2 There is only one possible meaning in each statement, and that meaning will be understood by any participant in the interaction in the same way.
3 There is no negotiation or co-construction of meaning.
4 There is no interaction between the interpreter and the other parties (communication is limited to language switching).
5 There is no interaction between the monolingual parties other than through the interpreter (i.e. gaze, gestures and body language are not considered key elements to any message).
6 Interpreting as a form of communication is not a situated practice (i.e. bound by the context in which it takes place).
7 Interpreting can be immune to social and cultural factors brought to bear by the interpreters and the two other interlocutors (i.e. participants' backgrounds are not accounted for in communication).

These issues can be seen represented in Figure 7.1 below.

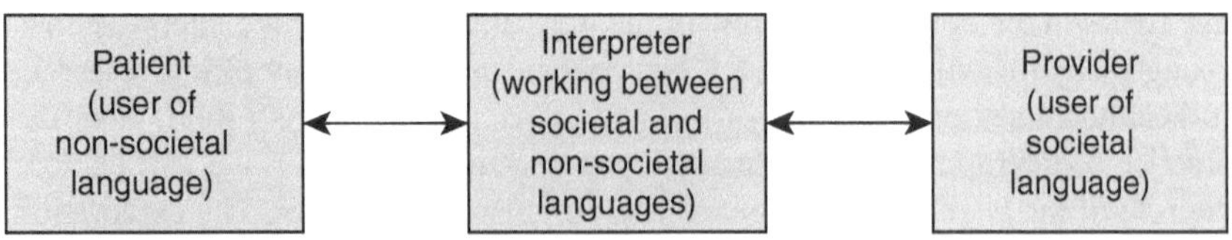

Figure 7.1 The invisible interpreter

Source: Adapted from Angelelli (2004a: 10).

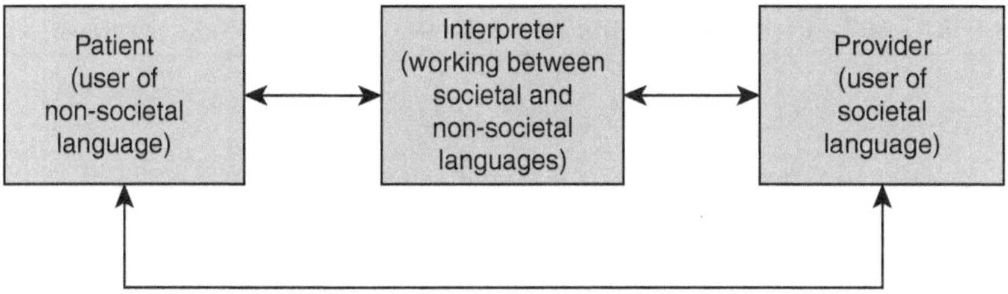

Figure 7.2 The interpreter as co-participant

Source: Adapted from Angelelli (2004a:10).

Research in interpreting intersecting with fields such as sociolinguistics, applied linguistics and sociology of language (e.g. Berk-Seligson 1990; Wadensjö 1998; Roy 2000; Angelelli 2004a, Baraldi and Gavioli 2012) portrays interpreters as essential partners to a cross-cultural conversation. This means that interpreters are not seen as conduits or modems but rather as co-participants in the interaction (Wadensjö 1998), taking turns talking, being addressed during talking (Roy 2000), facilitating, coordinating and controlling the traffic of communication in various PSI/liaison interpreting settings across languages (as also shown later by Baraldi and Gavioli 2012). This model (illustrated in Figure 7.2) highlights the interaction and the co-participation and coordination of the interpreter.

The results of the empirical research offer evidence of an interpreter who is a third co-participant rather than an invisible conduit; an interpreter who is a co-constructor in the interaction. Empirical research also helped understand what triggers interpreter's participation and what makes interpreters exercise their agency instead of remaining a conduit. The idea of treating interpreters as professionals whose performance cannot be impacted by factors such as their origin, gender, age or socio-economic status (as all human beings are) was intriguing. As evident by the results of further studies of interpreters' roles across settings using IPRI, (Interpreters Interpersonal Role Inventory – see page 156), the interpreter's interaction with other persons through the use of language cannot be immune to the interplay of social factors that impact any kind of interpersonal interaction through communication.

Figure 7.3 represents the visible model of the interpreter who exercises agency, which is highly complex. It builds on the fact that interpreting does not happen in a social vacuum. Rather, the interpreted communicative event happens in an institution which is itself permeable to societal norms and cultural blueprints. In addition, all parties to the interpreted communicative event (including the interpreter) bring with them their social baggage (age, ethnicity, gender, power, race, socio-economic status, solidarity) and their awareness of other participants' social factors. As discussed in Chapter 3, many of the behaviors interpreters exhibit are triggered by their views of others' social factors.

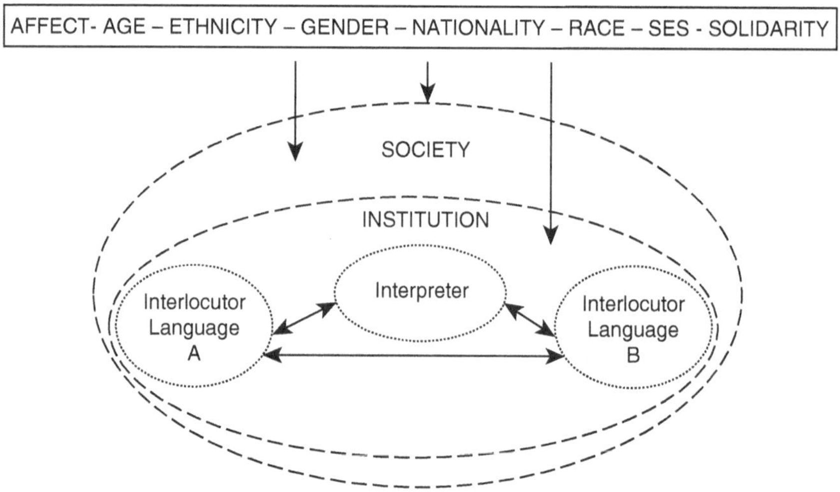

Figure 7.3 The visible interpreter who exercises agency
Source: Angelelli (2001, 2004a).

Even when professional ideology may portray an invisible interpreter, the study of the interpreters' perceptions and attitudes offers different evidence from an impartial and neutral presence. The study investigated whether or not the interpreters' own social factors (gender, age, ethnicity, socio-economic status, education) could in fact trigger or predict some of the interpreter's perceptions of the interpersonal role. Results of the study demonstrated that not all interpreters perceive their role in the same way and that their perception is linked to interpreters' background factors and the settings in which they work. In other words, female or male interpreters, younger or older interpreters and more or less educated interpreters perceive their roles differently and behave differently (with more or less empathy, exercising more or less power or solidarity, etc.) in all settings where they work.

Moreover, interpreters themselves do not consider their role as deprived of agency, as invisible, in any of the settings where they work (Angelelli 2004b: 76). This means that to a smaller or greater extent, they perceive that they play a role in building trust, facilitating mutual respect, communicating affect as well as message, explaining cultural gaps, controlling the communication flow and aligning with one of the parties to the interaction in which they participate. Angelelli also demonstrated that visibility (agency) is not a monolithic concept. The way in which interpreters exercise their agency (their power) varies according to the situated practice in which they are immersed. Role is fluid and can vary along a continuum within the same interaction, even within the same turn of talk, and has an impact on the exchange of information between healthcare provider and patient, through the interpreter.

Visibility by text ownership	Strategies for doing text ownership	Impact of text ownership on medical/personal information
High	Replacing the monolingual interlocutor	Highly consequential
	Alignment/Affect	
	Brokering cultural references	
	Expressing solidarity/exercising power	
	Expanding/summarizing	
	Exploring answers	
	Sliding up and down the register scale	
	Controlling the flow of traffic	
Low	<Openings/closings/positioning of self>	Inconsequential/ Highly ritualized

Figure 7.4 The visibility continuum at California Hope

Source: Angelelli (2004a:78).

This means that interpreters working in a public or private encounter have more or less flexibility to exercise their own agency (cf. a court room or a conference debate, a medical encounter or a teacher/parent conference) (Angelelli 2004b: 88–89). Participants in fact varied in how they perceived their role according to the setting where they worked. Medical interpreters perceived themselves as more visible than court or conference interpreters (Ibid.: 72–73). We discuss more about medical interpreter's roles and visibility in the next section.

A brief review of empirical studies on the role of healthcare interpreters

The role of HIs has been studied in different areas of the world, with different methods, language combinations and for different purposes. In Australia, research based on 13 interpreter-mediated consultations discusses the importance of what occurs at the end of the consultation, when the doctor summarizes their findings and recommendations (Tebble 1999, 2003). Because the ability of the doctor and patient to achieve rapport within this stage has a bearing on patient compliance (1999: 185–186), it is noted that "it is up to the medical interpreter to live up to the interpreters' code of ethics and convey what is said accurately." This statement seems to suggest that accuracy involves conveying the way in which information is expressed. In other words, accuracy refers to how the message is conveyed rather than to conveying the exact same content. Tebble uses excerpts from two authentic (videotaped) interactions to illustrate this issue, particularly how slight changes can actually change the message in a significant way. For example, one doctor tells a patient he has "high blood pressure," which is interpreted as "a little raised blood pressure" (1999: 193–194), potentially minimizing the seriousness of the issue.

In 2010 Angelelli and Slatyer administered the Interpreter Interpersonal Role Inventory (discussed above) in Australia. They also used mixed methods as in addition to the survey they conducted interviews, observations and focus groups to explore healthcare interpreters' perceptions and beliefs about their role. In French-speaking Switzerland, Leanza's comprehensive study on interpreters' role was conducted in interpreter-mediated pediatric consultations. Data for this study included participant observations, videotaped authentic consultations, and "stimulated recall" interviews with both interpreters and physicians. Participants were eight pediatric residents (seven female, one male) and four interpreters (three female, one male; three Albanians, one Tamil; three trained, one untrained). During interviews, Leanza finds that the physicians tended to refer to interpreters as translators (i.e. as invisible, but biomedically oriented translation instruments) (2005: 176). He also notes that physicians reported a loss of control in interpreter-mediated consultations, and they felt that communication was more difficult when an interpreter was involved (2005: 176). Two physicians mentioned an additional interpreter role, which is as a support for families outside of the institution (i.e. doing informal follow-ups in the community) (2005: 177). Interviews were also conducted with two of the four interpreters; they described themselves as performing a variety of roles. These included the role of supporting the family (as the two physicians mentioned above), the role of a host (helping make the family feel comfortable in the institutional setting, taking the lead in making introductions), translators, cultural informants (though only in the direction of physician to patient) and the role of bilingual professional, especially around nutritional issues (not clear what this entails) (2005: 178–179). In terms of the authentic data, Leanza analyzed the role of interpreters by focusing on how they positioned themselves during educational topics such as nutrition or sleep (he focused on how active/passive interpreters were).

In total, Leanza examined 187 interpreter utterances and coded 167 as translator/active translator, with the other 20 encompassing bilingual professional, monolingual professional, and cultural informant (2005: 184). Examples are given, from the authentic data, of interpreters positioning themselves as bilingual professionals (giving medical opinion) and cultural informants (explaining to physician about cultural practices that pertain to information given by a parent) (2005: 182–183). Leanza's work added two additional roles (active translator and monolingual professional) to Jalbert's typology of roles, which discussed five different options:

1 The interpreter as (active) translator: the interpreter minimizes her presence as much as possible. In this role the interpreter simply facilitates the communication process, not interfering with that the speakers say.

2 The interpreter as a cultural informant: the interpreter helps the healthcare provider to better understand the patient. In this role, the interpreter uses her knowledge of cultural norms and values.
3 The interpreter as a cultural broker or cultural mediator: the interpreter is a cultural informant but also a negotiator between two conflicting value systems or symbolic universes. In this role, the Cultural Broker needs to enlarge, provide explanations or synthesize healthcare providers' and patients' utterances to help both parties arrive at a meaningful shared model (of care, of behavior, etc.).
4 The interpreter as an advocate: in a value conflict situation, the interpreter may choose to defend the patient against the institution.
5 The interpreter as a bilingual (and monolingual) professional: the interpreter becomes the healthcare professional. She leads the interview in the patient's language and then reports to the healthcare provider. The interpreter can do this because of prior training in healthcare, or in a more limited way because of her knowledge of institutional practices and routines.

(Jalbert 1998 in Leanza 2005: 170)

For Leanza, "active translator" encompasses clarification of medical information (2005: 180) and "monolingual professional" as engaging in professional talk with the physician, displaying one's own health knowledge (2005: 181). He also recommends that interpreter training should explore all of these roles, and furthermore that medical professionals should be trained to work with interpreters (2005: 187). In his conclusions about this typology, Leanza states that except for the role of "translator" (in which interpreters attempt to be invisible), all other roles require the interpreter to align or identify either with the institution for whom they work ("bilingual professional") or with the community within which they work ("cultural informant," "cultural broker," "advocate") (2005: 170–171).

Leanza proposes a new typology of interpreter roles. In his view, community interpreters as cultural mediators are agents at four different levels (Ibid.: 186):

- Linguistic agent: acting as translator (+/− active).
- Community agent: acting as a cultural informant, cultural broker and as an advocate.
- System agent: acting as a bilingual professional.
- Integration agent: acting as welcoming support/follow-up staff member.

Community (PSI) interpreters have many cultural bridging roles beyond the straightforward task of translation from one language to another and vice versa, and this has not traditionally been acknowledged within biomedical literature. Leanza states that impartiality is not possible, nor even desirable, because "not only is cultural knowledge needed, but experiences of migration and with the receiving country's institutions are necessary for professional community interpreting practice" (2005: 171). The aim of Leanza's study, therefore, was to explore the roles of medical interpreters in detail, by looking at both authentic interpreter-mediated interaction data and the perceptions (though interviews) of medical practitioners and interpreters themselves.

In the United States, and based on a case study conducted over six months in a public hospital between Spanish-speaking patients and English-speaking providers, Davidson (1998) proposes a new model of turn taking in interpreter-mediated interaction and illustrates its application to interpreter-mediated medical discourse. His model is based on the idea of "common ground" – the shared understanding that participants in a conversation work to achieve. As a conversation develops, the shared understanding between participants grows. Davidson's aim was to create a model that would better account for interpreter participation than more traditional, and perhaps overly simplistic, models that view the interpreter as a conduit (or an "overhearer" rather than a "participant"). According to Davidson, interpreters cannot possibly be viewed as conduits, because "in order to negotiate and capture the meaning of an utterance produced within an ongoing discourse, one must be a participant in the discourse itself" (2002: 1275). Interpreters who are not acknowledged or allowed participant status therefore are unlikely to be able to understand and interpret the interaction successfully. Another reason he claims traditional models are inaccurate is that they allow no space for interpreters to use agency (cf. Angelelli 2004a, 2004b), for example in clarifying information; if the interpreter cannot clarify information (cf. Roy 2000; Baraldi and Gavioli 2012), then this common ground becomes even less achievable (2002: 1282).

Contributing to this line of research, and to understand (1) how interpreters perceive their agency, their roles as healthcare interpreters (2) how they act out their role in practice and speak about their agency, their visibility, in their own words, Angelelli (2004a) added two dimensions to the study of interpreters' role in a medical setting: (1) the dimension of social factors impacting communication and (2) the dimension of ethnography to the study of role, accounting for (a) the perceptions of role (using psychometrics in 2004b), (b) the materialization of role in practice and (c) the reflection about it. Her work focused on first exploring interpreters' own beliefs about their roles and behaviors in practice through IPRI. The goal of this exploration was to understand how/if interpreters' own background and social factors (age, gender, ethnicity, socio-economic status, level of education, etc.), in addition to the medical setting, shape interpreters' self-perception of their roles. Second, she added to the body of knowledge of medical interpreting the dimension of extensive and intensive data collection and sustainability throughout time. She conducted an ethnography of a medical interpreting service which involved 22 months of observations of healthcare interpreters at work in a public hospital in California. A total of 392 interpreted communicative events were observed, transcribed and analyzed. The role medical interpreters play, their role shifts and the way in which interpreters go about doing their job, their interactions with others, their routine and their ways of speaking – all can be observed in detail in a prolonged period of time without any manipulation by the researcher of the participants or of the site itself. This is called naturalistic data. Sustained observations throughout time in real environments (compared to an experimental situation or a role-play) afford the researcher to find typicality and gain reassurance about competing explanations for the same phenomenon. This can be achieved because patterns of behaviors begin to emerge only throughout repeated naturalistic observations throughout time.

Also in the United States, focusing on signed language interpreting, Swabey and Mickelson (2008) discuss challenges of interpreter role definition, particularly with regard to professional organizations (and their codes of ethics), interpreter training and legislation. They take a "systems" approach to this discussion (i.e. they view the profession as a system, from those individuals and organizations who comprise the system to outside systems that have an impact on it). According to Swabey and Mickelson, over the years, various legislative acts prohibiting discrimination have been passed (e.g. the Americans with Disabilities Act 1990). This has brought interpreting into new settings and has challenged interpreters to examine and redefine their professional role (2008: 56). The role of sign language interpreters in a medical setting has been challenged previously by Metzger (1999).

Empirical research has contributed significantly to our understanding of role, first, by embracing a continuum of possibilities when describing it rather than reducing it to a dichotomy, and second, by the ways in which role has been studied. This means, for example, embracing scientific empirical work and moving away from theoretical assumptions and prescriptions. Empirical work can provide unequivocal evidence of a continuum of roles interpreters can take on as they position themselves in an interpreted communicative event. This means interpreters are a lot more than a conceptual dichotomy (e.g. neutral or advocate), and they can be studied using a variety of methods. Results of empirical research at times permeate professional practice and at other times they do not. This accounts for the variability of prescriptive and descriptive discourse that we can see in codes of professional practice. Sometimes a tension emerges between theoretical assumptions, resulting in prescriptive rules, and empirical research, resulting in descriptive statements.

Views emerging from discussions in professional associations

The concept of role has been at the core of professionalization and professional associations rules and regulations as a result of ongoing discussions among HIs about their experience in practice and the behaviors prescribed by their professional associations. Initially, discussions were about only the extreme positions, such as those of a neutral or active interpreter. In the United States (the first country to have medical/healthcare interpreting associations and short courses/training sessions for healthcare interpreters), the dialogue began in 1994 at a conference on (spoken language) healthcare interpreting in Seattle and was continued through a series of working meetings over the following six years. Discussions centered around the scope of the healthcare interpreter's role as well as the nature of the interpreter's relationship with clients, and participants in the meetings had some very different (polarized) views on these issues. Two opposing perspectives of the role of the healthcare interpreter emerged from the early discussions: the neutral interpreter and the active interpreter. The neutral interpreter perspective views the interpreter as an instrument who should not engage with or create any kind of relationship with other participants, and who is concerned only with passing messages from one language into another and vice versa (Beltran-Avery 2001: 4). In contrast, the active interpreter perspective views interpreters as "socially present" individuals who are often a part of the patient's culture. It recognizes that participants' (including the interpreter's) age, gender and cultural backgrounds can affect interaction, and that the interpreter sometimes needs to intervene to alert participants to cultural misunderstandings or to assist participants in achieving mutual understanding (2001: 4). These discussions were happening at the same time as the results of empirical research conducted in California (Davidson 1998; Angelelli 2001) were showing unequivocally how communication is never immune to the interplay of social factors.

This group became aware that there were more "conceptualizations" of the healthcare interpreter's role out in the field than a simple dichotomy of neutral versus active. Four different "conceptualizations" along a continuum (from neutral to active) began to be considered:

1 *The interpreter as conduit.* The main responsibility of the interpreter as conduit is the transmission of messages. This perspective is in line with the notion of neutrality. This perspective does recognize that cultural background information can help an interpreter to better achieve equivalency of meaning. However, any kind of "cultural brokering" (including clarifying information) is seen as risky behavior for the interpreter. It should be the responsibility of the provider and should be requested by them.
2 *The interpreter as manager of the cross-cultural/cross-language mediated clinical encounter.* This perspective acknowledges that the very presence of an interpreter will change the dynamics within a medical encounter. Each participant brings their own expertise to the encounter, and the interpreter is seen as an active participant with linguistic/socio-cultural expertise in their own right. In order to main the flow of communication, the interpreter can actively assist when necessary to bridge cultural gaps. It is recognized that the interpreter is the only one in the encounter who has access to every utterance. This is understood as a powerful position. The group suggests "it is the responsibility of the interpreter to use her power in the interest of the health care goal" (Beltran-Avery 2001: 8).
3 *The incremental intervention model.* This perspective sees the interpreter as flexible in their role, and depending on the demands of the situation, the interpreter can be a conduit, a cultural broker or at the most "intrusive" level, an advocate. It is important that the interpreter is transparent in any choices she makes (Ibid.: 9). Within this view, since the power dynamics between the patient and provider naturally favor the provider, neutrality is perceived as "detrimental to advancing the goal of the encounter" and, therefore, not serving anyone's interests (Ibid.: 9). This interpretation of power dynamics and its alteration is problematic.

4 *The interpreter as embedded in her cultural-linguistic community.* This perspective assumes that "the person performing the function is there as a whole person embedded in the social fabric of her community" (Ibid.: 10). A fact that has been established in research seemed difficult to accept by a professional organization. It recognizes that the act of interpreting cannot be separated from the interpreter's linguistic and cultural background, from their relationship to the other participants, or from institutional and socio-political contextual factors. This approach is often favored by small communities and First Nations communities, where interpreters must be credible members of the community (Ibid.: 10). These people often hold more than one position outside the community, so a nurse or a social worker, for example, may act as an interpreter also. Beltran-Avery explains that transparency is crucial when an interpreter assumes different roles in order to maintain trust (Ibid.: 10).

This white paper finishes with some "cautious agreements" about the role of the healthcare interpreter. These agreements acknowledge that interpreters must sometimes be active in order to achieve accuracy and to facilitate shared understanding, although they also warn that these actions must be transparent and that the overall goal is always the well-being of the patient (Beltran-Avery 2001: 12–13). However, the conclusion the group arrived at was not to agree on a fixed definition of the healthcare interpreter but to acknowledge that all perspectives are useful and to encourage ongoing dialogue between stakeholders. Beltran-Avery describes a "creative tension" between the two extremes of the continuum, concluding:

> The conduit perspective keeps the field grounded in the central function of the interpreter – the linguistic conversion that allows communication between a patient and provider who do not speak the same language. The embeddedness perspective challenges the profession to consider its place in a holistic view of the patient's well being, a wholeness of heart, mind and spirit. One without the other is incomplete.
>
> (Beltran-Avery 2001: 14)

At the same time as this discussion was going on, another healthcare professional organization also in the United States, the California Healthcare Interpreting Association (CHIA), published *The California Standards for Healthcare Interpreters: Ethical Principles, Protocols and Guidance on Roles and Interventions* (CHIA 2002). These standards have been in use in California since the fall of 2002. The standards document is groundbreaking in the sense that it is not a set of theoretical assumptions and is not prescriptive in tone. Instead, it is empirically based, it is grounded in medical ethics and it presents an ethical decision-making model to resolve ethical dilemmas faced by interpreters (see Chapter 8). In addition, guidance is provided on four common medical interpreting roles and on the extensive feedback process developed for validating the standards by interpreters across California.

Of interest to us in this chapter are the four roles described by CHIA as a continuum of possibilities. The first role discussed in the standards is "Message converter" (Davidson 2002: 36).

> It involves facilitating the flow of the conversation between two parties. The second role of "message clarifier" includes gaining more information from a speaker to transparently explain a message or concept in an alternate or more easily understood manner to facilitate communication. The third role, "cultural clarifier," involves transparently confirming and providing cultural information, particularly about cultural health beliefs. "Transparency" is defined in the CHIA glossary as,
>
>> the idea that the interpreter keeps both parties in the interpreting session fully informed of what is happening, who is speaking, and what the interpreter is doing. . . . Whenever interpreters intervene by voicing their own thoughts and not the interpreted words of one of their clients, it is critical that they ensure that a) the message is conveyed to all parties and b) everyone is aware that the message originates from the interpreter.
>
> The fourth role, "patient advocate" – a prohibited role for the court interpreter – may be required in the healthcare setting to support the health and well-being of the patient.
>
> (Davidson 2002: 38–41)

> The CHIA standards, firmly grounded on empirical research, acknowledge that the role of the interpreter is multifaceted and that the interpreter shifts between different roles within an interaction. Sometimes the boundaries are porous. CHIA clearly states that interpreters play multiple roles in addition to the message converter role portrayed in earlier writings. Including the patient's advocacy role as part of a continuum has not come without controversy. "Unlike normal service activities, such as directing the patient to the pharmacy, advocacy might include helping ensure the patient gets the benefit of an interpreter on their next visit, or identifying the basic right to an interpreter for either the patient or the clinician. CHIA recommends that interpreters intervene as little as necessary to allow the two monolingual interlocutors to resolve their differences once a misunderstanding has been drawn to their attention. But, as stated by Kontrimas (2000: 4),'Interpreters cannot and should not be responsible for everything that everyone does, or doesn't do. But, if they happen to notice something starting to go wrong, it is reasonable to bring it to the attention of someone who can correct it before it becomes a problem, rather than sit back and watch a disaster unfold.'"
>
> (Angelelli, Agger-Gupta, Green and Okahara 2007)

Clearly, the patient advocate is a demanding role, and it is neither encouraged nor forbidden by CHIA. It calls for significant experience, judgment and confidence on the part of the interpreter. It has consequences, and interpreters need to be aware of them. It involves potential invasiveness, controversy and risk, both for the patient and for the interpreter. This is the reason behind CHIA recommending this role as an optional one. The decision to intervene as a patient advocate must be left to the interpreter's judgment as a healthcare professional. For some readers/interpreters, this degree of latitude in a document that regulates a profession may be new, but it is not unusual in other professions. Given that most professionals conduct their work by what Mintzberg describes as the "standardization of skills," precise directions and prescriptions are unnecessary because training and ethics establish a known set of skills (1993, 1983: 4–6).

Interpreting, as we have discussed before, is a situated practice. Therefore, role cannot be considered in abstract and defined as one size fits all. There is not one single descriptor that will fit all types of roles HIs play as they go about doing their work. Therefore, it is imperative we see the difference between a top-down and a bottom-up approach to role and come to terms with a descriptive rather than a prescriptive approach. Role is not monolithic; it is multifaceted. Role is dynamic and cannot and should not be boxed in one set of rules. It depends on the communicative event, which as we have seen in Chapter 1, has various components and participants who bring intentions, goals, social factors and so forth. Roles vary across settings, across interpreted communicative events and within them. Studies conducted on role have shown how interpreters shift roles within the same interaction according to communicative needs.

Role explained by metaphors

When interpreters discuss their work (whether they interpret between spoken or signed languages), they sometimes resort to metaphors to explain their work. In several studies researchers have interviewed interpreters to understand their own views on their role and have explored the use of metaphors. The most common ones are:

Interpreters as

- *Bridges*: Interpreters think of themselves as bridges, as a bridge between languages and cultures. "My role is just to be a bridge, a bridge between the doctor and the patient" (Hsieh 2009: 140). This metaphor has been used not only by interpreters themselves but also by professional associations in their newsletters and by company in their advertisements.
- *Multi-purpose bridges*: When doctors ask a question that, in their experience requires a yes/no answer, such as "Does it hurt or doesn't it?" (Angelelli 2004a: 87, Elda), but the patient does not answer the question directly and instead engages in telling a story, the interpreter is not only bridging languages or cultures but also ways of speaking. And the interpreter intervenes to refocus the patient so that the provider can get the answer needed to proceed. In this case, Elda stated, "*A ver señora María, por qué no me dice si le duele o no asi yo le contesto la pregunta*?" [Let's see Ms. Maria, why don't

you tell me if it hurts or it doesn't so that I can answer the question?]. In this way, the interpreter is not just a bridge, as having no agency other than being there and transferring words/meanings across; the interpreter is present and actively engaging the patient, playing a role to obtain the type of information needed (Ibid.: 130).

- *Detectives*: When doctors ask questions about medical history, such as "Any chronic illnesses running in the family?" or "Have you ever been hospitalized or operated on?" some interpreters decide to investigate the full range of possibilities rather than simply asking a question and taking the answer at face value. So, for example, if a patient is an immigrant or has been displaced, the interpreter, when exploring these questions of hospitalization or surgery, may add to the patient a reference to place of origin and place of residence such as "here or there" or "this country or your country" (Angelelli 2004 a). They also do this exploration with medicine intake. If providers ask, "Are you taking any medicine now?" using their knowledge about how medicine works in other areas, interpreters may say: "have you ever taken any medicine, medicine sold over the counter, prescribed, or any remedy given to you by *la comadre* (Godmother) Juana." By doing this, once again, interpreters believe they cover all possible ranges of possible answers.
- *Diamond connoisseurs* (Angelelli 2004a: 131): At times, providers need specific answers, such as yes/no. They need relevant, clear and brief answers. Patients may not always give relevant short answers. Instead they may engage in storytelling that may contain relevant, less relevant or completely irrelevant information. So, when a patient answers a yes/no question with a story, the patient opens up a bag with stones, diamonds and dirt. In this metaphor, the diamonds represent the crucial pieces of information that the interpreter needs for the interview to succeed; the stones represent the irrelevant pieces of information and the dirt is the discourse that glues all the pieces together. The interpreter must be capable to distinguish diamonds from ordinary stones. This is a big responsibility. The interpreter must also keep all the stones and the dirt handy because he never knows when those pieces will become relevant during the interview. What may look like an ordinary stone at a certain point may become a diamond later on as the interview unfolds.
- *Mine diggers* (Angelelli 2004a: 131–132): Patients vary in their sense of cooperation and their willingness to participate. Therefore, interpreters need to be able to access information. They must find a way to dig for it until they can uncover the information they need. In this sense, interpreters are like mine diggers. They continue to excavate until they reach what they need to reach. What makes a strategic interpreter is to know how to ask the same question in different ways until the necessary information is obtained.
- *Voice machine, robot*: "If you want to keep your job, you want to become, really, a kind of robot in order to keep your job. . . we are like the voice, we are not a person" (Hsieh 2009: 139).

Perceptions of healthcare interpreters' role

Interpreters as perceived by HO administrators or managers

During observations performed at private hospitals in tourist destinations in Spain (Angelelli 2015), professional interpreters hired as staff members of private organizations (providing among other services in medical tourism) were expected to attend to the foreign patients' medical and administrative needs, to be in constant communication with the foreign patient and their family and even to take phone calls form the service-unit manager while conducting another interpreting assignment. Being on duty constantly and facing interruptions during other interpreting assignments increases stress levels for staff interpreters.

In a private medical clinic in Southern Spain, one interpreter who was fluent in five European languages and had been working for a long time as a medical interpreter in that clinic, was constantly under pressure as she was supposed to answer the phone from the clinic dispatcher about other requests for her work in other units of the clinic as she was in the middle of interpreting for a patient and a doctor (Ibid.).

The interpreter's whole day was spent running from one floor to another, but this is what she had to do to satisfy her boss (the clinic administrator). The interpreter was highly regarded and very professional. She was, however, asked to work in impossible conditions. As one can see, many interpreters find themselves between a rock and a hard place. They are reprimanded by the physician/provider with whom they are working when they are interrupted to assist a foreign patient and, at the same time, and they are reprimanded by the service-unit manager for not responding immediately when they are called on their mobile. It goes without saying that these constant interruptions were not appreciated by the patient or his family.

During interviews with these interpreter staff members immediately after the field observations, we learned that high levels of stress and burnout are not uncommon among healthcare interpreters in this organization and that stress accounted for big turnover in the position of staff interpreters. As a consequence, in this organization the administration was convinced that it would be better to hire bilingual employees rather than professional interpreters. In reality, interpreters were working under unnecessary pressure because the HO was hiring bilingual staff that could not engage in simultaneous or consecutive interpreting, as expected by HO. They did not have the skills. So, instead, bilingual staff answered the phone, gave directions and helped orient new patients to the organization in one or more of the languages they used to communicate. However, when interpreting was required for the patient to communicate with a healthcare provider, the bilingual employees at the reception desk did not interpret. They directed these requests to the staff interpreters, who were already spread extremely thin.

Healthcare interpreters' perceptions of their own role

Focusing on a Mandarin-speaking population in the Midwest United States, Hsieh (2009) explored how healthcare interpreters conceptualize their role by shadowing two Mandarin/English interpreters and observing and audio-recording encounters in which they interpreted. She conducted interviews with 21 medical interpreters (representing a wide range of cultural and language backgrounds) and five managers (p. 137). According to Hsieh, 21 out of 26 interviewees identified with the "non-thinking" conduit model of interpreting, however from the descriptions there is no clear differentiation of the 21 being all the interpreters participating or a mix of interpreters and managers. She notes, "without seeming to be aware that these behaviors require them to become an active participant in the communication" (p. 141)

Interpreters liked the conduit role (at least, what they perceived it to be) because they thought it enabled a complete transfer of information while also reinforcing provider-patient relationships. With regard to the complete transfer of information, Hsieh gives transcript examples from her authentic data, of interpreters accurately conveying both linguistic and nonlinguistic (i.e. pointing, tone, volume) information. In terms of reinforcing relationships between participants, Hsieh explains that the conduit role appeals because it creates the illusion of a dyadic interaction. Interpreters in Hsieh's authentic data used many strategies to facilitate better provider-patient relationships, for example using first person, changing comments or questions directed at the interpreter into comments or questions for the other participant, positioning themselves behind the speakers, making minimal eye contact and so forth (pp. 146–148). She claims that this is evidence that interpreters use specific and conscious communicative strategies and are not "non-thinking" conduits at all: "although interpreters in this study demonstrated their desire to accomplish the communicative *goals* of a conduit role, these goals were not accomplished through a conduit *role*" (pp. 149–150).

Also in the United States, during Angelelli's ethnographic study of Spanish-English interpreters at California Hope (2004a), she captured the following example. It shows how interpreters reflect on their role while breaking bad news to family during a medical interview:

Tape 604 Julio turns 113, 115, 117

JULIO: "*Son los casos que son difíciles, ¿no? de comunicar. A veces, ahí es donde, donde llega uno a hacer algo. . . más de puente si tú quieres. . . porque pues a veces, el profesional está tan acostumbrado a dar malas noticias que. . . no toma el tiempo, o el tacto para informarlas ¿no? Y es ahí cuando uno debe decir. . . tome asiento por favor, o sea, de que sabe que. . . su papá falleció. Este, y así es donde tienes que tener tacto. O sea, poco a poco ¿no? Como estábamos creo yo, en nuestra cultura acostumbrados de que no nada más es, sabes qué. . .*"

[These are the cases that are difficult, to communicate, right? Sometimes, and that's where, where one has to do something. . . more like be a bridge if you want. . . because sometimes, the healthcare provider is so used to giving bad news that. . . he does not take the time, or the care to give bad news properly, right? And that's when one should say to the person. . . take a seat please, you need to know that. . . your father passed away.so. and it is in saying this that one has to be tactful. Do it, little by little, right? As we are, I think, used to in our culture. . . we are used to not just. . . you know what.]

INTERVIEWER: *¿Los doctores aprecian eso? ¿Entienden eso? ¿O esperan que lo hagan?*

[Do doctors appreciate this way (of breaking news)? Do they understand it? Or do they expect you to break the news and be done with it?]

JULIO: "*Algunos. . . algunos. . . algunos no. Algunos ni se dan por enterados. Este, algunos se asombran, este, otros se espantan, porque es un hecho, es como es, y, ¿no?, el hecho de morir, de la muerte, pues todos nos vamos a morir. Pero, eso ninguno lo esperamos, ¿no?. Este, un caso en particular, llegó un familiar, trayendo un paciente de México, que volaron aquí, llegando el avión, este, falleció. Entonces lo trajeron aquí, pero pues. . . ya. . . lo trataron de resucitar, este, llegó y el doctor le dijo, no pues para el ni modo, ya venía muerto. Hicimos lo que pudimos, pero pues falleció. ¿Te imaginas tú? La familia, venían como cinco mujeres, trayéndolo desde México, ¿no? O sea, el esfuerzo que hicieron de. . . aunque los doctores de allá les dijeron que no estaba bien que volara, el esfuerzo de ellos de tratar de salvarlo, de subirlo a un avión, este, aunque estaba enfermo este pariente, la paz de traerlo aquí para que de alguna manera buscara una mejoría, ¿no? Y tan fácil como que se murió. . . ¿no? claro que estas mujeres empezaron a pegar gritos en un cuartito así de. . . tan chiquito como este. . . ¿no?, y se espantó el doctor, ¿no? Pero, era algo que. . . o sea, no lo puedes nada más decir así como lo dije. Y aunque tratas de. . . poco a poquito ir, este, tuvieron una reacción de asombro para. . . para un estadounidense.*"

[Some, some. . . some do not. Some do not even know. . . or care about these differences. Well, some are surprised by these differences, others are frightened, because. . . for them death is a fact dying is a fact. . . it is what it is. . . we are all going to die. But, that nobody expects, right? In this case, in particular, a patient's relative came, bringing the patient from Mexico, they flew over here, when the plane landed he died. So they brought him here, but then. . . they tried to resuscitate him and the doctor said. . . for him there was nothing we could do, he was already dead. We did what we could, but he died. Can you imagine? The family, five women came, bringing him from Mexico, right? This is the effort they made. . . although the doctors over there told them that it would not be good for him to fly, they made this huge effort to try to save him, to get him on a plane, well, although this relative was sick, the peace of mind they got for bringing him over here so that he would somehow be better, right? And the news was broken as plainly as he died, that simple. . . right? Of course these women started screaming in a tiny little room. . . as small as this one ok?, And the doctor got scared by the screaming. But, it was something that . . . I mean, one cannot break this news just like I did. And although one tries to say it gently. . . little by little they had a reaction that was unexpected for an American.]

Healthcare providers' perceptions of the role of healthcare interpreters

Providers' perceptions about the role that HIs play in the interactions vary considerably (from helpers, to tools, to colleagues, to a participant that they can or cannot trust). These perceptions have been documented in studies. Providers' perceptions differ from patients' perspectives and they also differ according to the interpreter's employment status (i.e. interpreters hired to perform as interpreters, as full time members of staff, interpreters working for agency in charge of provision, freelancers working on site, freelancers working remotely (whether using telephone or video)).

While some healthcare providers see interpreters as necessary to do their work with a linguistically diverse population, they express concern about working with interpreters who may go beyond the interpreting role (Singy and Guex 2005). Their study was conducted in French-speaking Switzerland and was based on questionnaires (medical practitioners only but over 650 each time, two rounds, 12 months apart), focus groups (also two rounds, approximately 15 participants in each, including patients, interpreters and medical professionals), and 35 semi-structured interviews with immigrant patients (2005: 47). Based on reported data, the way different participants in an interpreter-mediated medical interaction conceptualize the interpreter's role was studied. Data was collected between 1998 and 2001 and coincided with the training of "ICMs" (interpreting cultural mediators).

Many practitioners (psychiatrists and nurses) interviewed in Switzerland showed what the authors call a "naïve" view of interpreting. On the one hand, participants valued the work of interpreters and thought they were necessary, but they were wary of interpreters going beyond their perceived conduit role. Participants were worried interpreters might not interpret everything, or that they might add advice of their own (2005: 47–48). Some healthcare practitioners viewed interpreters as active participants, but the overriding view was that an interpreter is a "walking bilingual dictionary" (2005: 48) or described as a translation machine (Leanza 2005). Other studies have also shown healthcare providers at times relinquishing control of the medical interview to interpreters on the guise that interpreters know the culture better, understand facial expressions and so forth (Angelelli 2004a; Hsieh 2009).

Whether interpreters are perceived by providers as tools, for their own use, for example, to keep the patient on track, to find out information, to give them cultural tips, to take medical history, to look at facial expression and body language during EKG, delegating control of the medical interview (Angelelli 2004a; Davidson 2000, 2002; Hsieh 2016: 206–214), the issue becomes one of trust and teamwork. Do providers trust interpreters? (Hsieh 2016: 217–229). Do they see them as a member of the healthcare team? A teamwork approach seems to be at odds with the perception of the interpreter as a tool to be used for one's own purpose. There is at times a possible mismatch between interpreters' and healthcare providers' expectations. Whether intentional or not, it is a fact that a third participant in the interaction influences behaviors, content and so forth (Hill and Zepeda 1992). In addition, interaction is based on shared understanding, so interpreters who are not afforded participant status would not be able to understand and interpret the discourse.

Patient's/family members'/friends' perceptions on the role of healthcare interpreters

As reported in several studies (Davidson 2000; Angelelli 2004a; Hsieh 2009), because interpreters share a language and cultural views with the patient, it is not uncommon for the patient to think of the interpreter as the party with whom understanding can be constructed, the party to be trusted, the partner in the conversation. Immigrant patients view interpreters not only as necessary for meaningful communication, but also as active participants as they work to ensure both language and culture are understood (Singy and Guex 2005: 49). This perception can be explained by the term "positionality of the interpreter" as "a unique social and cultural position relative to the communities within which they work. It is they who are positioned 'between worlds' and who make possible communication with 'outsiders'" (Cokley 2009: 1). Positionality has been studied in spoken languages on those who provide access to others in terms of acculturation or access to services (see, e.g., the work on Latino immigrants to the United States by Orellana 2009; Valdes et al. 2000). Even when for sign language users the interpreter has always been considered as the link, the connection with the "others," the non-signers, positionality as such began to be used in spoken languages, and the term was not used in sign languages in the early 2000s.

The intricacies of role

As we have seen throughout this chapter, the interpreters' role has been a preoccupation for researchers, professional organizations and interpreters. Some of the issues discussed above have been studied systematically while others have only begun to be explored. Studies on the role of healthcare interpreters have produced different types and sizes of data in one language combination or across languages.

In all of the studies, however, an unresolved tension continues to transpire through the issues highlighted. The tension is about reality and prescription. The reality of the roles, the responsibilities, the expectations and job requirements of healthcare interpreters in their workplace, the intricacies of interpreting as a situated practice and theoretical assumptions about those roles, responsibilities, job requirements and expectations. The interpreter's role, like roles in general, is not monolithic. As demonstrated by research on the role(s) of interpreters across the various settings where interpreters work, several dimensions are included in the interpreter's role. Some are related to the self (self-perceptions of behaviors, beliefs); others result from the interaction with the participants and the various perceptions and expectations each of the participants have about the role of the interpreter; and other dimensions arise from the context where interpreting happens (i.e. the micro context, the local and physical one in which the encounter takes place, the pressures from various working practices and constraints and the macro one involving the dimension of more than one culture interacting, more than one worldview). Figure 7.5 illustrates four dimensions of the interpreter's role already studied (Angelelli 2004b: 52).

Personal/Interpersonal (concept of self)	Socio-cultural (situational/contextual)
Self in Social Relations	Cross-cultural

Figure 7.5 Four dimensions of interpreters' role

Source: Angelelli (2004b: 52).

In addition to role being multidimensional and multifaceted, role is played out in interaction. In her study about interpreting as interaction, Wadensjö argues that talk is different from text and it is a result of interaction. Therefore, expecting a linear and literal rendition from an interpreter may not be feasible. There is of course the exception of, for example, a cognitive evaluation in a neurological/psychiatric consultation or an expert witness testimony in a court of law. These are just two examples of communicative events, when the form of expression is as important (if not more) as the content. Wadensjö describes a taxonomy of interpreters' renditions (1998: 104–108) and clearly shows what the interpreter may do in order to accomplish a communicative action. The interpreter may omit, add, rephrase or may provide divergent renditions, close renditions, substitute renditions and so forth.

A taxonomy of interpreter's strategies used in medical interviews results from the ethnographic study conducted at California Hope discussed above (Angelelli 2004a: 78). Based on 392 provider-patient interpreted communicative events in a medical setting recorded during 22 months, it shows a continuum of strategies used by interpreters (from introduction of self, to register shifts, to replacing monolingual interlocutors, etc.) that increasingly impact the personal and technical information relayed. Angelelli also sheds light on many of the social factors that lead participating interpreters to make certain decisions, such as to explain things differently to patients (e.g. "because patients cannot understand technical jargon," or "because doctors speak about pain in scales and patient do not"; 2004a).

The value of scientific studies, the value of empirical research and the value of supporting claims with evidence is what differentiates ideology from knowledge and what gives credibility to studies and positions. We then ask ourselves the question, how is role taught and learned? It is not feasible to anticipate all the issues that may arise during interpreted communicative events and all the different roles the interpreter can play, or the behaviors they can exhibit. Based on existing research reports, we can (and we should) gain a thorough understanding of the inventory of behaviors that have been identified. We can reflect on the fact that these behaviors (like any others in life) have consequences. While each interpreting communicative event is unique, while interpreting is a situated practice, there are boundaries that need to be considered when it comes to playing the role of an interpreter, a provider and so forth.

It is imperative that we reconcile the tension between expectations and reality of role so that interpreters can in fact do their jobs without feeling they cannot measure up to expectations. So, after reading about role, it becomes clear that the tension between the actual demands of interpreters' workplace and the statements about what is the appropriate or acceptable role of the healthcare interpreter and what is not, which role is desirable, ethical or feasible and which one is not (we elaborate more on ethics in Chapter 8) needs to be resolved. This is why we need to engage with professional associations, bring research and practice together, revisit codes of ethics and understand the difference between aspirations, attainable goals and learned behaviors that can be adopted (Angelelli 2007; Dysart-Gale 2005; Hsieh 2009) in the situated practice of healthcare interpreting.

B. Research, observe and reflect

Go to Chapter 6 and look at the transcript presented in section B. The transcript is between a female doctor and a male patient and it is interpreted by Marta. We will do another reading of the transcript, and this time, we will focus only on the role of the interpreter.

We will look at the turns Marta interprets and see, in its context, what kind of role Marta is playing. Remember role is not static, and interpreters may shift roles in the same interaction several times. Role shifts can occur between turns of talk as well as within the same turn of talk.

As we re-read, let's focus also on what we have learned in this chapter. Are any of the metaphors discussed in this chapter applicable to her role? If so, which turns would be evidence of this?

Now, choose two turns of talk in which Marta acted, either as prescribed by the code of ethics (you can use the one from your area/country or turn to Chapter 8 for examples) or by deviating from it (she may have deviated just a little or too much). Based on the turns you chose, and what we learned in this chapter, analyze the consequences of renditions, focus on how/if the way Marta interpreted affected the communicative goals of the participants and impacted on communication and on her responsibility as an interpreter and interlocutor.

C. Journal writing

In this chapter we have discussed different issues surrounding the role of the healthcare interpreter. Reflect on the different views that the participants have about the interpreter, their expectations of the healthcare interpreter, their communicative needs and so forth. Think about how the role of the healthcare interpreter has changed throughout time and how it has evolved. Put role in the context of professionalization of healthcare interpreting (discussed in Chapter 1). Think of the differences and similarities between a mediator and an interpreter. Based on your work experience, on your experience as a member of a linguistic community, and what you have read in this chapter and beyond, how would you describe your role? Which of the models discussed (those described in professional association codes, or learned from research on interpreters showing what interpreters do when they work, how they talk about their role, the metaphors they use or what they think about it) reflects better what you do everyday as you interpret. Why? Think of the responsibilities and consequences of taking or not taking certain roles described by professional associations. Justify your responses.

D. Further tasks

This is a segment of an encounter between a genetic nurse and a pregnant woman, Ramira, who comes to the visit in her second month of pregnancy. We have heard about their interaction in Chapter 6 (Further Tasks).

The nurse has explained to her that the amniocentesis procedure is an option patients have, not a required test. She also explained to Ramira that healthcare providers need to present patients with their options. Ramira did not want to hear about the tests earlier in the encounter because she has mentioned previously to the interpreter (who interpreted the information to the provider) that she is determined to have her baby. The clash of needs, beliefs and expectations caused some misunderstanding.

We come in as the encounter is closing and the interpreter and the patient are having this side conversation. The patient is asking the interpreter to explain once again to the provider that she really does not want to hear about the procedure because she does not want to have it. And that she is grateful for the possibility but she does not want it.

Read this segment and reflect on the role of the interpreter. After reading, discuss the questions below.

138 P *Pero. . . mire. . . yo. . . yo quiero que usted le explique. . . verdad. . . que yo no tengo hijo*
but, listen I, I want you to explain to her that, true, that I do not have children

139 I *aja*
aha

140 P *ni un hijo*
not even one child

141 I *aja*
aha

142 P *entonces es el primer hijo. . . y si se me llega a lograr*
so this is my first child and if I can have the baby

143 I *aja*
aha

144 P *vamos a ver. . . que a mi me salga mal mi bebé. . . esteeemmm. . .*
let's see. . . and if my baby is not right ehmm

145 I *es su bebé, ¿verdad?*
it is your baby, right?

146 P *aja. . . en ese caso. . . ¿qué es lo que pueden hacer?*
aha, in that case what can they do?
147 I *Sí. . . yo se. . . y va a tener que. . . determinar. . .*
yes, I know. . . and. . . you will have to determine. . .
148 P *Aja. . . o sea si me sale mal. . . ¿me lo sacaría?*
aha, I mean if the test results are bad, would I get rid of the baby?
149 I *Le darían a usted para decidir si sí o no. . .*
they would ask you to decide if yes or no
150 P *No. . . pero no me lo sacaría yo. . .*
no, but I would not get rid of the baby
151 I *Entiendo. . . y por eso le dije que no tenia que estar ahi. . . hablando más. . . pero. . . ya sabe. . . yo nada más soy una intérprete. . . ¿Me permite un momentito, eh?*
I understand, and that is why I told her that she did not have to continue speaking about this, but, you know, I am only an interpreter. Excuse me for a minute, okay?
152 P *Sí*
yes

Read each of the turns carefully looking at what the interpreter does with the form and content of the talk. In which turns (if any) is the interpreter showing evidence the following:

1 Turn ____: being a co-conversationalist.
2 Turn ____: answering for the participants (taking their role).
3 Turn ____: being professional.
4 Turn ____: being compassionate.
5 Turn ____: showing empathy.
6 Turn ____: not being professional.
7 Turn ____: helping the parties by establishing mutual respect or trust.
8 Turn ____: aligning more with one party than the other.
9 Turn ____: justifying or judging the other party.

Point to the turns of talk in the transcript where you can see the interpreter having any of these behaviors. You can also find more and add them to the list.

References

Americans with Disability Act of 1990 (as amended). Available at www.ada.gov/pubs/adastatute08.htm (Last accessed April 2, 2018).

Angelelli, C. (2015). *A study on public service translation in cross-border healthcare: Technical report*. Luxembourg: Publications Office of the European Union. ISBN 978-92-79-47163-6.

———. (2007). Validating professional standards and codes: Challenges and opportunities. *Interpreting: International Journal of Research and Practice in Interpreting*, *8*(2), 175–193.

———. (2004a). *Medical interpreting and cross-cultural communication.* London: Cambridge University Press.

———. (2004b). *Re-visiting the interpreter's role.* Amsterdam: John Benjamins.

———. (2001). *Deconstructing the invisible interpreter: A study of the interpersonal role of the interpreter in a cross- linguistic/cultural communicative event.* Ph.D. diss., Stanford University, Stanford, CA.

Angelelli, C. V., Agger-Gupta, N., Green, C., & Okahara, L. (2007). The California standards for healthcare interpreters: Ethical principles, protocols and guidance on roles and intervention. In C. Wadensjö, B. Dimitrova, & A.-L. Nilsson (Eds.), *The critical link 4: The professionalization of interpreting in the community* (pp. 167–180). Amsterdam and Philadelphia: John Benjamins.

Baraldi, C., & Gavioli, L. (Eds.). (2012). *Coordinating participation in dialogue interpreting.* Amsterdam: Benjamins, pp. 251–268.

Beltran-Avery, M.-P. (2001). *The role of the healthcare interpreter: An evolving dialogue.* Available at www.ncihc.org

Berk-Seligson, S. (1990). *The bilingual courtroom: Court interpreters in the judicial process.* Chicago: Chicago University Press.

CHIA (California Healthcare Interpreters Association) (2002). California standards for healthcare interpreters: Ethical principles, protocols, and guidance on roles and intervention. Sacramento: California Endowment.

Cokley, D. (2009). Shifting positionality: A critical examination of the turning point in the relationship of interpreters and the deaf community. In M. Marschark, R. Peterson, & E. A. Winston (Eds.), *Perspectives on deafness: Sign language interpreting and interpreter education: Directions for research and practice* (pp. 3–28). New York, NY: Oxford University Press.

Davidson, B. (2002). A model for the construction of conversational common ground in interpreted discourse. *Journal of Pragmatics, 34,* 1273–1300.

———. (2000). The interpreter as institutional gatekeeper: The social-linguistic role of interpreters in Spanish-English medical discourse. *Journal of Sociolinguistics, 4,* 379–405.

———. (1998). *Interpreting medical discourse: A study of cross-linguistic communication in the hospital clinic.* Ph.D. diss. Stanford University, Stanford, CA.

Dysart-Gale, D. (2005). Clinicians and medical interpreters: Negotiating culturally appropriate care for patients with limited English ability. *Family and Community Health, 30*(3), 237–246.

Hill, J., & Zepeda, O. (1992). Mrs. Patricio's trouble: The distribution of responsibility in an account of personal experience. In J. Hill & J. Irvine (Eds.), *Responsibility and evidence in oral discourse* (pp. 197–226). Cambridge: Cambridge University Press.

Hsieh, E. (2016). *Bilingual healthcare communication: Working with interpreters in cross-cultural care.* New York and London: Routledge/Taylor and Francis Group.

———. (2009). Bilingual health communication: Medical interpreters' construction of a mediator role. In D. Brashers & D. Goldsmith (Eds.), *Communicating to manage health and illness* (pp. 135–160). New York: Routledge.

Leanza, Y. (2005). Roles of community interpreters in pediatrics as seen by interpreters, physicians and researchers. *Interpreting, 7,* 167–192.

Metzger, M. (1999). *Sign language interpreting: Deconstructing the myth of neutrality.* Washington, DC: Gallaudet University Press, 216 pp.

Mintzberg, H. (1993, 1983). *Structure in fives: Designing effective organizations.* Englewood Cliffs, NJ: Prentice-Hall, pp. 4–6.

Orellana, M. F. (2009). *Translating childhoods: Immigrant youth, languages, and culture*. New Brunswick, NJ: Rutgers University Press.

Reddy, M. J. (1979). The conduit metaphor: A case of frame conflict in our language about language. In A. Ortony (Ed.), *Metaphor and thought* (pp. 164–201). New York, NY: Cambridge University Press.

Roy, C. (2000). *Interpreting as a discourse process*. Oxford: Oxford University Press.

Seleskovitch, D., & Lederer, M. (1984). *Interpreter pour traduire [Interpreting to translate]*. Paris: Didier erudition, 311 pp.

Singy, P., & Guex, P. (2005). The interpreter's role with immigrant patients: Contrasted points of view. *Communication and Medicine*, *2*(1), 45–51.

Swabey, L., & Mickelson, P. (2008). Role definition. In C. V. Garcés & A. Martin (Eds.), *Crossing borders in community interpreting* (pp. 51–80). Amsterdam and Philadelphia: John Benjamins Publishing Company.

Tebble, H. (2003). Training doctors to work effectively with interpreters. In B. Louise, G. Bastin, I. Hemlin, & H. Clarke (Eds.), *The critical link 3: Interpreters in the community* (pp. 81–95). Amsterdam: John Benjamins.

———. (1999). The tenor of consultant physicians: Implications for medical interpreting. *The Translator*, *5*(2), 179–200.

Valdes, G., Chavez, C., & Angelelli, C. V. (2000). Bilingualism from another perspective: The case of young interpreters from immigrant communities. In A. Roca (Ed.), *Research on Spanish in the United States: Linguistic issues and challenges: Chapter 2* (pp. 42–81). Somerville, MA: Cascadilla Press.

Wadensjö, C. (1998). *Interpreting as interaction*. New York: Addison Wesley Longman Inc.

Further readings

Angelelli, C. V. (2014). "Uh. . . . I'm not understanding you at all": Constructing (mis) understanding in provider/patient-interpreted medical encounters. In B. Nicodemus & M. Metzger (Eds.), *Investigations in healthcare interpreting*. Gallaudet Studies in Interpreting (pp. 1–31). Washington, DC: Gallaudet University Press.

Biagini, M., Boyd, M. S., & Monacelli, C. (Eds.). (2017). *The changing role of the interpreter: Contextualising norms, ethics and quality standards*. New York and Abingdon: Routledge, 264 pp.

Grbić, N. (2010). "Boundary work" as a concept for studying professionalization processes in the interpreting field. *Translation and Interpreting Studies*, Special issue: *Profession, identity and status: Translators and interpreters as an occupational group, Part 2: Questions of role and identity*. M. Shlesinger & R. Sela-Sheffy (Eds.), *5*(1), 109–123.

Mason, I., & Ren, W. (2014). Power in face-to-face interpreting events. In C. V. Angelelli (Ed.), *The Sociological Turn in Translation and Interpreting Studies* (pp. 115–133). Amsterdam and Philadelphia: John Benjaimins.

Tyulenev, S. (2016). Agency and role. In C. V. Angelelli & B. J. Baer (Eds.), *Researching Translation and Interpreting* (pp. 17–31). New York and Abingdon: Routledge

Varela Salinas, M. J., & Meyer, B. (Eds.). (2015). *Translating and interpreting healthcare discourses/Traducir e interpretar en el ámbito sanitario*. Berlin: Frank & Timme, 368 pp.

8 Ethics in interpreter-mediated medical communication

Goals

In this chapter we will:

- Explore the difference between personal and professional ethics.
- Learn about ethics of healthcare interpreting in your geographical area and beyond.
- Learn about ethics of other professionals working with healthcare interpreters.
- Reflect about ethics and responsibilities of freelancers and staff interpreters.

Learning outcomes

By successfully completing this chapter, readers will be able to:

- Compare and contrast ethical principles of various professionals working with healthcare interpreters.
- Identify ethical issues and dilemmas.
- Analyze an ethical issue and dilemma.
- Apply a decision-making process to an ethical dilemma.

Before discussing ethics in healthcare interpreting, it is important to discuss ethics in general and distinguish between personal and professional ethics. Ethics are central to decision-making. Decision-making can be about personal or business matters; it can be made by only one person or by a group of people. When discussing personal ethics, we generally refer to moral issues and behaviors, which tend to be classified as right or wrong. When professionals use their skills and knowledge to serve the public, they may encounter problems that may turned into a moral issue. It is when these moral issues arise and when professionals turn to ethics for guidance to analyze and resolve these issues that professional rather than personal ethics comes into play. Thus, when personal and corporate ethics come together, we shift from personal ethics to professional ethics. Issues, however, as we have encountered throughout the book, are complex and do not always lend themselves to be so easily compartmentalized. This chapter is about professional ethics. Professionals, through their education and professional practice, have acquired knowledge and skills. By applying these, they can make informed decisions. These decisions generally cannot be made by the public at large. In this chapter, we will discuss the ethics of all the professional groups that come together during the interpreted communicative event in a healthcare encounter and focus specifically on how the healthcare interpreter navigates the different layers of self and others' professional ethics.

A. Professional ethics surrounding healthcare interpreting

As we have seen throughout this book, interpreting is a situated practice and interpreted communicative events occur within social and physical contexts. In this situated practice, various layers of ethical principles interrelate. Participants in interpreted communicative events, regardless of their role (whether they are healthcare providers, administrators, interpreters or cultural mediators), observe their own professional ethics. These specific professional ethics may converge, diverge or be at odds with each other. This is a reality. Therefore, interpreters need to be aware of competing principles, expectations, roles and responsibilities and place their own ethics in this context. It is misleading to believe that it is enough for interpreters to understand their own code of conduct and the ethical principles that guide their practice. This is important and basic knowledge professional interpreters must have. Interpreters, however, represent one professional group that comes together in contact with other professional groups as represented in Figure 8.1.

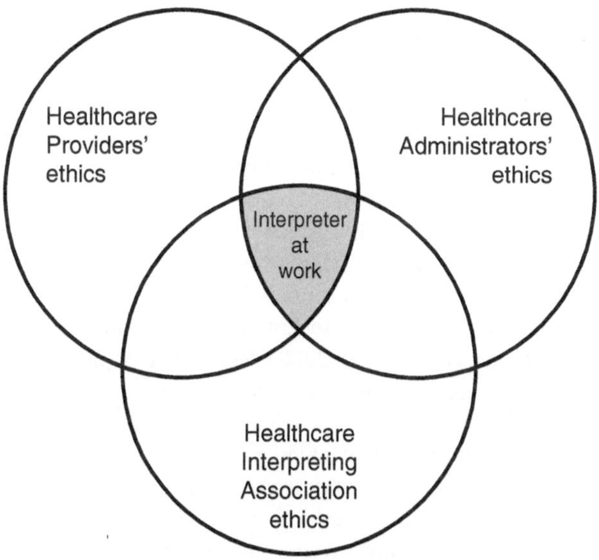

Figure 8.1 Intersecting ethics at work

Ethics of physicians

In the settings where healthcare providers work, one well recognized code of professional ethics is the one by which medical doctors abide. It is also known as the Hippocratic Oath. Held sacred by physicians, it is one of the oldest binding documents and the earliest expression of ethics in the Western world. New physicians swear to uphold specific ethical standards, which include the principles of medical confidentiality and non-maleficence. The term "medical ethics" was first used in the early 1800s. An English author and physician, Percival, published a document describing expectations and requirements of medical professionals working in medical facilities. There are several documents that constitute the basic pillars of medical ethics, among them the Nuremberg Code (1947) and the Declaration of Helsinki (1964). Medical ethics is based on four main pillars: (1) patient autonomy (i.e. does one, as the professional, show respect for the patient and allow the patient to make an informed decision?); (2) non-maleficence (i.e. does one's own behavior harm the patient?); (3) justice (are there consequences of one's own behavior to the wider community?); and (4) beneficence (does one's own behavior benefit the patient?). The observation of medical ethics is widely accepted and practiced throughout the world (Riddick 2003). This does not mean, however that there is consistency across countries or that there are no issues (Hlavac 2010). Many times, issues are related to how medical doctors communicate/do not communicate with linguistically diverse patients. This is a clear example of complex practices and borderlines among professional groups coming together for the well-being of the patient. This issue of communication begs the question of ethics that may go beyond medical doctors' behaviors to include healthcare organizations and healthcare interpreters as well.

As we have seen in this book, issues reported by interpreters to social workers, or the office of patient advocacy in a healthcare organization, for example, as well as research produced in the fields of healthcare, health communication, health literacy and interpreting studies (to name a few fields of inquiry as examples), shed light on these problems of communication between doctor and patient. They also highlight the fact that when patients do not have access to the societal language, they do not get the full benefits of a doctor/patient interaction. Studies on healthcare provision to linguistically diverse patients in domestic violence in the United States, for example, unequivocally show that when patients seek care and they do not speak the societal language, not being able to communicate is a major source of isolation and an obstacle to seeking healthcare and help for Latina and Asian immigrant women (Bauer et al. 2000). Research comparing the benefits of palliative care among English-speaking and non-English-speaking populations in Australia indicates that non-English-speaking patients may receive less optimal palliative care than fluent English-speaking patients (Chan and Woodruff 1999). In a study focusing on errors in pediatric consultations produced by professional and non-professional interpreters working in healthcare organizations, results indicate that errors in medical interpreting in the pediatric setting are common and have potential clinical consequences (Flores et al 2003). Ad hoc interpreters are more likely to make errors that can lead to clinical consequences.

This is an illustration of how issues can be complex and how responsible behavior on the part of the team is required. So, when/if issues arise because others step into the role of professional interpreters because the latter are either not brought into the interaction or not available, whose responsibility is it? The healthcare organization's? The medical doctor's? The bilingual employee's (nurse, lab technician, cook, janitor)? The friend's or family member's, who stepped in as asked? Or is it the responsibility of all parties involved? One thing is certain: it is not solely the responsibility of the bilingual person who tried to/was told to perform.

Ethics of nurses

In addition to physicians, another professional group with whom interpreters frequently work are nurses. The professional ethics of nurses also interact with the ethics of interpreters. In a study conducted in a nursing care management unit (Rassin 2008), professional and personal values of 323 Israeli nurses were measured to identify which factors affect 20 professional and 36 personal values. The professional values rated the highest were human dignity, equality among patients and prevention of suffering. The values that ranked in the top ten were all those related to nurses' responsibilities toward patients. Confidentiality and altruism were not highly rated. In regard to personal values, honesty, responsibility and intelligence were rated first. This study reports significant differences among personal and professional values. These differences are attributed to culture, education, professional seniority, position and field of expertise.

In the example above, discussing the involvement of non-professional interpreters, if a nurse is called upon to interpret on the basis of her bilingualism or even worse, on the basis of her family name (Cambridge 1999), and the nurse is not an interpreter, then the professional ethics of the nurse and the healthcare organization could be called into question. And the ethical dilemma always appears to be, what is indeed better, or what is the lesser of two evils: no interpreter and no (or basic) communication, or a non-professional interpreter and the likelihood of taking a risk of getting a message across inappropriately? In this case, the dilemma is really for the nurse, the physician and the HO, as they abide by a code of ethics that clearly has the well-being of the patient at its core. This should not be a dilemma for family members or friends who, in addition to worrying for their loved one, step up to the plate on the basis of a relationship with the patient and are not bound by professional ethics. However, as we have seen throughout the book (especially Chapters 1 and 3), none of these issues is to be taken lightly as there are several and opposite outcomes/consequences to actions taken.

Ethics of healthcare administrators and managers

In terms of ethics of HO administration and management, for example, in some healthcare systems that have recently experienced important political, social and economic changes (e.g. countries that have gained independence from the former Soviet Union and joined the EU more recently) (see Bankauskaite and Jakusovaite 2006), problems have been identified. These problems, mostly related to lack of trust in the system and in providers, suggest the need to broaden the conceptual understanding of ethics in healthcare and focus on ethics management to tackle ethical problems in countries in transition. The most salient ethical problems reported in the administrative sector in Lithuania, for example, are related to (1) the healthcare reform process (e.g. health inequalities, inadequate access to services and lack of trust in the healthcare system) and (2) interprofessional relationships (e.g. communication with and cooperation among healthcare and social workers) (Bankauskaite and Jakusovaite 2006).

A similar study conducted in Bulgaria reports the most salient issues are the lack of transparency in the reform process and paternalistic attitudes from healthcare providers (in general, beyond administrators) to patients. This means that providers not always consider the personal values of patients, their financial responsibilities and lifestyle. Consequently, as the population is not appropriately informed, the population does not understand the reason behind a particular change/reform and why certain decisions related to their healthcare have been made. Among issues requiring attention, it is worth mentioning the informal payments for legally free healthcare. The World Health Organization (WHO) Regional Office for Europe outlined three main values as the ethical background for public healthcare: (1) health as a fundamental human right; (2) justice and solidarity among countries, groups and sexes; and (3) participation of people, groups, communities, institutions, organizations and sectors in the process of healthcare promotion (Health21 1999). It is particularly important to think of upholding these values in the context of a diverse population as the one we currently see in many parts of the world. If the WHO stipulates health to be considered a fundamental right of humans, but at the same time, access to healthcare is not feasible because of a difference in languages that can simply be solved with healthcare interpreters, then how can this ethical principle and main value be upheld? And what does this mean for healthcare administrators and providers? And, for the purposes of this book, what does this mean for healthcare interpreters? What is a healthcare interpreter supposed to do, and what can a healthcare interpreter do?

Ethics of interpreters

Unlike a monolingual medical event, in an interpreter-mediated medical event, in addition to patients, healthcare providers and administrators, there are also the parties that represent language services. Providers of language services, be they healthcare interpreters hired as staff members, freelance interpreters working for an agency or agency providers themselves, have to follow their own set of ethical guidelines, principles or standards of practice. These are the principles that guide the provision of healthcare interpreting services rather than the provision of healthcare. Sometimes healthcare organizations may not be aware, for example, of the differences in responsibilities and expectations between interpreters and healthcare providers/administrators, or even between interpreters and cultural mediators. So, in addition to observing their own professional ethics as well as those of others, healthcare interpreters many times engage in client education to make sure clients (the healthcare administrator, the provider or the patient) understand their role and responsibilities.

Providers have different opinions regarding the interpreter's duties and responsibilities. For some, the interpreter is a tool that they can use to accomplish their communicative goals; for others, the interpreter is a necessary evil. When providers are interviewed about their work with interpreters, many times they refer to interpreters as their allies. In their writings on the views of interpreters, Hsieh and Kramer (2012) discuss the tensions, challenges and dangers of considering the interpreter as a tool. In their study, some providers report that they prefer professional interpreters to family members because professional interpreters are hired to work for them. Providers also expect professional interpreters to be the ones that know how to redirect the patients so that they focus on the answers required rather than engaging in providing irrelevant information that takes a long time (Davidson 2000). Providers also have stated preferring family members to professional interpreters because the family members have more information on the patients and can offer providers more background information that they say can be helpful for them (Angelelli 2015). These differences between providers' views and expectations of the interpreters' roles and responsibilities can be a source of stress for interpreters. The more the parties to the interpreted communicative event understand what interpreters can and cannot do, or are supposed to do or not do, the more manageable and less stressful the job of the interpreter becomes.

A review of the ethical principles guiding healthcare interpreter's professional performance reveals no standardization across specific associations in the world, although many share similar values. Even when HI does not have a universal code of ethics, as apparently is the case with the medical profession, many of the basic principles of professionalism seem to be shared in various HI codes (e.g. CHIA 2002; HIN 2004; IMIA 2006; NCIHC 2004; NRPSI 2016). Among those are:

- Exhibiting a professional demeanor.
- Demonstrating respect for persons.
- Showing no preference or bias toward either party involved in the interaction.
- Recognizing own limitations of competence (linguistic, subject matter or emotional).
- Refusing jobs for which one believes one is not qualified.
- Maintaining impartiality.
- Keeping confidentiality, except if disclosure of information is detrimental to safety of persons, or is required by law.
- Disclosing any real or perceived conflict of interest.
- Keeping up to date with one's professional development and professional requirements.

This sharing of values paves the way to standardization. This seems to be a characteristic of professions moving from emerging to established. Currently there are efforts at the ISO level to develop specific guidelines for medical interpreting. The status of this profession varies across countries. There are countries in which associations of healthcare interpreters do not exist and no provisions are made for healthcare interpreting, even when the practice exists in the country (e.g. Korea,

Thailand and other countries in Asia, where there is a significant amount of medical tourism and language brokering occurs). On the other end of the continuum, there are countries with healthcare interpreting associations at the national and state/provincial level (e.g. Australia, Canada, United States). Several member states in the European Union do not have a code of healthcare interpreting per se (e.g. Germany, Greece, Italy, even when there is mobility of EU patients traveling under Directive 2011/24/EU or Regulation (EC) 883/2004). Other member states have guidelines/ethical principles for interpreters working in the public services in general (i.e. Spain, UK), and still others have legislation regulating the job of the cultural mediator and no provisions for interpreters (e.g. Italy).

When professional associations for healthcare interpreting get established, they generally start by adopting a code of ethics. To do this, a writing group is appointed. Having a code of ethics appears to be considered one validating sign of a profession. It is important, however, to have a deep understanding of the purpose of the code of ethics. Especially in healthcare interpreting, codes of ethics or standards of practice have been conceptualized differently. For some organizations they may be as a set of values shared by a profession, an aspiration, a teaching tool, a certification tool and/or a tool for monitoring performance (e.g. AUSIT 2012; CHIA 2002; HIN 2004 in Abraham et al.; IMIA 2006; NCIHC 2004; NRPSI 2016). In addition, codes of ethics can be theoretically or empirically based. A theoretically based code may establish principles that are agreed upon by members of the organization. Ideally this would occur in consultation with all members. Many times it is the members who can afford to sit around the table and take the time to work on a code, its conceptualization and authorship who end up shaping its content and also carrying the responsibility for it. Those members may be funded to do this work or they may be volunteers for the organization. Alternatively, when a code of ethics is empirically based, it is informed by research in the field and takes into consideration the specificity of the situated practice as well as the changes of the practice throughout time. In addition to basing a code in empirical findings or in theoretical assumptions, some organizations validate their code of ethics with research conducted among their own members (e.g. CHIA 2002 and in Angelelli 2007b; NCIHC 2004).

In addition, codes of ethics and professional organizations views of them change over time (Ko 2006). The history of the RID (Registry of Interpreters for the Deaf) in the United States is an example of a shift that occurred over years. The RID moved from a prescriptive, rule-based code to ethics toward a rights/values-based code of professional conduct (Swabey and Mickelson 2008: 57–61). They then discuss interpreter training, particularly a lack of consistency in terms of standards, and a lack of clarity about what best practice actually is and what that means for interpreter role definition, as discussed in Chapter 7.

Examples of intersecting ethics

Various professional groups coexist in a healthcare setting and each bring in their specific professional ethics. Members of these groups may come together in a medical interview, which the interpreter may be called upon to facilitate. Therefore, in an interpreted communicative event, several ethics intersect. At times, issues may arise that may require a broader view, a more interdisciplinary conceptualization of ethics. At other times, issues may be very narrow, specific and clearly falling under one specific set of ethical principles (e.g. related to appointment management or the interpreter's skills). When multiple sets of ethics come together, and a clash of ethics occurs, or when conflicting views arise from different standpoints, which one prevails? Can one set of professional ethical principles actually prevail over others? What is the healthcare interpreter supposed to do? What dilemmas may arise for interpreters during an interpreted communicative event? And, do the other participants in the event know and understand the ethical principles to which interpreters abide? More often than not, interpreters have to learn about the ethics of the medical profession, the healthcare administration and others. This learning is part of the interpreter's general education and preparation for an assignment. The other participants may not know about interpreters' roles or responsibilities. In fact, many times the other participants' expectations of what interpreters should or should not do may not match what interpreters, in fact, can or cannot do.

Ethical dilemmas faced by interpreters and decision-making processes

Let's consider a common example presented to participants in ethical workshops which has been discussed extensively in the literature of healthcare interpreting: several interpreters' codes of ethics prescribe that interpreters should not interact with client/patients without the presence of the provider or the other interlocutor. Most healthcare interpreters, however, report to encounter the opposite in their place of work, so they perceive a tension between a rule at their own place of work and a rule in the code of ethics of the professional association to which they belong. Interpreters learn to avoid being alone with the patient, as this may be misleading for the patient, who may find in the interpreter a companion, a co-conversationalist. Interpreters, however, have reported how, in their place of work (i.e. a hospital), they are expected to accompany the patient to different areas in the hospital.

An example to illustrate this is the following: at the end of an encounter, if the doctor prescribes some medication to the patient, the interpreter may be asked to guide the patient from the doctor's office to the pharmacy. And if the patient cannot walk or is in a wheelchair, the interpreter may be expected to push the chair for the patient. This is a clear example of conflicting expectations that may pose an ethical dilemma to the interpreter. Interpreters need to be ready to explain why they can or cannot do something they are asked to do, and at the same time, they also have to consider the job description to which they have agreed. And, above all, interpreters are human beings and they may have their own personal ethics telling them to be kind and help or not to get involved. At the end of the day their contract is with the healthcare organization and interpreters need to learn how they manage personal and professional ethics with the mandates from their workplace. These are important considerations for interpreters and, at times, sources of conflict and stress. Meaningful conversations need to take place between service managers and interpreters to make sure all sets of ethics are respected and synchronized.

Another example of an ethical dilemma which is also discussed in the literature frequently is when patients address the interpreter directly to share information in confidence, to say things they may not want the doctor to know. This information could be in relation to the medication they take or do not take, the diet they observe or do not, or the exercise they should do or not do and so forth. As discussed before, there are different ways in which these issues are used.

Based on empirical data collected during a study in California among Hmong and Cantonese-speaking patients to measure bilinguals' readiness to work as healthcare interpreters, Angelelli designed a test to include a line from a patient that presented a dilemma to the interpreting test-takers (2007a). The patient was not taking the regular cholesterol medicine prescribed by the doctor. While discussing results, the doctor expressed his concern as they did not show any decrease in spite of the medication, which the doctor believed the patient was taking. As the doctor was expressing this concern and the interpreter was interpreting the information into Cantonese for the patient, the patient looked at the interpreter and did not react. When the doctor was at his computer station looking at previous records to compare cholesterol tests, the patient whispered the following to the interpreter in Cantonese: "Two times a day I take my herbs with hot water and I feel fine. I am not taking any of these pills. But, please don't tell this to the doctor." This situation happens quite often. In fact, a similar scenario was developed by the CHIA Standards and Certification Committee as an example of ethical dilemmas presented in the CHIA *Ethical Principles, Protocols and Guidance on Roles and Interventions* (CHIA 2002: 48–55).

The examples above illustrate some of the dilemmas interpreters confront as they do their work. In their own words, at times, interpreters feel as if they are trapped between a rock and a hard place. This occurs when the requirements of their place of work may be at odds with their role as prescribed in their professional code of ethics (Angelelli 2007a). When interpreters share a language with a patient, interpreters are often perceived by patients as their only link between them and the health system of the host country. It is not unusual to learn about patients providing unsolicited information to interpreters when they are not in the presence of the healthcare provider (e.g. in the waiting room waiting for an appointment) or while walking from point A to point B in the hospital (e.g. from the consultation room to the laboratory). Based on ethical guidelines, this situation creates an ethical dilemma for interpreters. What are they supposed to do with unsolicited information that may have consequences for the well-being of the patient? Should they keep it to themselves or take action to provide this information to the HCP, who may know if it should be used or not? Should they tell the provider and thus violate the patient's trust?

Since there are always consequences to actions, interpreters need to reflect on the issue at hand by following an ethical decision-making process and asking themselves six questions before acting or avoiding to take action (CHIA 2002).

These questions have different aims, which combined should help the interpreter in solving the ethical dilemma. The aims of the questions are the following:

1 Interpreter asks questions to determine if there is indeed a problem: this is done by exploring the issue further with the patient in order to determine patient's concerns and/or address patient's misconceptions.
2 If there is a problem, the interpreter clearly identifies it, states it and considers the ethical principles that may apply to the case. Once the principles are identified, the interpreter ranks them in order of applicability.
3 The interpreter then clarifies their own personal values that may relate to the problem at hand.
4 The interpreter then considers alternative actions (e.g. take action and tell the provider; take no action [i.e. do nothing] and not tell the provider) and weighs benefits and risks of taking or not taking action.
5 After a careful evaluation, the interpreter decides to carry out the actions chosen (e.g. tell or not tell the provider).
6 The interpreter evaluates and reflects on the outcome of their decision of taking or not taking action. By doing a thorough evaluative reflection, the interpreter learns from this experience what to do similarly/differently the next time a similar issue arises.

(adapted from CHIA 2002: 49)

In the following section, we will discuss several scenarios bringing together various professional groups and presenting issues of various types to explore the application of an ethical decision making process on the art of the interpreter to various situations.

B. Research, observe and reflect

In the following exercise we will focus on a case. As you read about it, write down the issues that in your opinion constitute ethical issues for each of the professional groups involved. Tease out the issues to see if they are related to the interaction of competing ethics, to intercultural differences between provider and patient, to differences in conceptualization of life or death, to differences in language and communication, to people's expectations of each other or all of the above.

The case in point is about a 75-year-old Muslim man who was critically ill and whose life has been sustained artificially since he had lost capacity (six months ago). This man has never issued a power of attorney or granted any advance decisions in regard to his health or personal welfare. After a series of discussion and evaluations, the medical team in charge of Mr. Haddad (fictitious name) felt that it was in the patient's best interest to limit treatment. Mr. Haddad's family disagreed, as family members felt that they knew their spouse/father better and would thus be in a better position to judge what their father would want. Mr. Haddad, who was indeed critically ill and has not responded to treatment in the last six months, was a devout Muslim. The family members found it very difficult to get sound advice about what was in the best interests of Mr. Haddad. For them, the need to reconcile and balance medical and religious viewpoints was key. When the family spoke to the imam or to Islamic scholars, they did not think they received enough information about when/where a line should be drawn. The family members explained how, in the Qur'an it is taught that for every life that is saved, the whole of mankind is saved, but if you take away life, it is as if you have killed all of mankind. Without any additional specialist advice, this presented an incredibly heavy burden on the family. So, as devout Muslims, they continued to do what they thought was the right thing – by asking the doctors to continue treatment. In Mr. Haddad's case, the doctors did follow the family's wishes, but it was repeated and emphasized several times to the group that in the absence of a document clearly stating Mr. Haddad's health or welfare advanced decisions (which generally is in the form of a power of attorney), the final decision would always be taken by the healthcare team. This notion of persons empowered to make decisions over the life of others was clearly not shared with Mr. Haddad's family or the Muslim community in the area. For many Muslims, it is generally the case that everything should be done to preserve life and then it should be left in God's hands to see if these treatments succeed or fail.

This case was presented in front of experts in the subject matter (faith and life decisions) during a workshop held in London. While many agreed with the resolution stated above, others believe that pain is given in this world to take away suffering in the next. Within the group attending the workshop, however, there were several different views. Some attendees stated that if a person is considered/diagnosed as brain dead then treatment should be withdrawn. It was agreed that if in doubt, individuals should consult their local imams for advice. However, as Mr. Haddad's family discovered, sometimes imams may not be qualified at the level required for these types of decisions/cases, or it may be really difficult to be able to access accurate information to make an informed decision. Not many imams have training from the Muslim faith in this area. It is therefore not surprising that Mr. Haddad's family were not able to find a clear-cut answer. We should not forget, however that the family was seeking and expecting an answer from the religious, not the scientific, domain.

Reflect on this case from the perspective of an interpreter. You could have been the interpreter in this case had the family not spoken the societal language. As you think of the situation and the issues, tease them out and do the following:

1 Brainstorm on the ethical issues and dilemmas from the perspective of the interpreter or posed to the interpreter. Draw a mind map.
2 Look at the mind map. Write down the issue, the tensions you see, and your reflections on them. All of these may influence how you do your work, and you have to make a decision. Your decision cannot be arbitrary. It needs to be justifiable and supported. Find support/justification for your decision in your code of ethics, in the intersection of multiple ethics and so forth. You can use the following table if you find it helpful.

Issue	*Tensions*	*Reflection*	*Decision to act*	*Support for decision*

C. Journal writing

Choose one of the three scenarios described above, or go back to the article on Syrian refugees in Chapter 1, or choose any experience you have had yourself or read about involving healthcare interpreting and an ethical issue. This will be the interpreted communicative event (ICE) in which the issue occurred. Reflecting on an empirical situation, an ICE will provide you with a context. Identify the ethical issues arising from the ICE. Then identify the code of ethics of your local association ("my code of ethics") or of one of the healthcare/medical interpreting associations across the world and read pertinent sections. You will run the issue you identified through the two codes of ethics. You will look for similarities and differences in how one issue can be analyzed, classified and so forth. In preparation for the entry, you can use this table to organize your thoughts and find support for your decisions:

Context of chosen issue	*Ethical issue(s) identified*	*My code of ethics*	*Another code of ethics*	*Comments*

By comparing and contrasting empirical issues and principles in codes of ethics, reflect on the profession of healthcare interpreting in general. Then consider the other professionals interacting with you, their ethics, expectations and so forth. Reflect on the clients, the patient and the patient's family and their personal ethics and expectations.

In your entry, focus on thoughts about the interaction of personal and professional ethics and expectations of parties for whom you work as well as the ethics and expectations of the professional healthcare interpreter.

D. Further tasks

Professional groups coming together in an interpreted communicative event: different or similar professional ethics?

To understand if the interpreter's ethics align with another professional's ethics, we look at different scenarios and how each of the participants in an interpreted communicative event may react as a result of applying their own professional ethics, which may or may not align with each other.

The following three **scenarios** take place at a **public hospital** in an **urban area** of your country. They all are examples of conflicting ethics or ethical dilemmas which interpreters face frequently. The issues presented are authentic and have been collected during fieldwork observing medical interpreters. They have been transcribed and now adapted to fit this exercise.

- Your first task before working with each scenario is to fill the contextual information that would help you situate this interaction in a place where you see yourself working/observing.
- The setting, both physical and social, should make sense to you in your political, geographical, social and economic context.
- Remember that interpreting is a **situated practice**.
- As you get ready to reflect on these scenarios, also consider the following:
    - If you, as the interpreter, are working as a freelancer, a staff member in a healthcare organization of your area, or if you work for an agency or for the government. Based on your status, you may have to take a different action.
    - What the linguistic minorities in your area are, and specifically the one for which you generally interpret given your language combination (XX). Ask yourself the following questions: What do you know about this minority group in your area (are they immigrants, political refugees? A mix? Have they been displaced? Do they come individually? In family groups? In waves? What was their area of origin (e.g. have they all come from a same region or country)? What linguistic/cultural variations can be found among them? What information do you have about their cultural/religious beliefs, festivities and so forth?
    - Which is the societal language (YY) in your area? Is there one or more? What is the relationship between the societal language and the languages of the linguistic group(s) for whom you interpret?
- Take a moment to reflect on all of these issues and fill in the blanks with data. Contextualizing will allow you to reflect on your reactions to the following scenarios in a more realistic way.

Scenario 1: You are called to interpret between a medical intern in psychiatry and a depressed patient who has refused psychiatric treatment. The patient is a middle-aged male. He is of XX origin. He is fluent in XX but speaks almost no YY, thus the need to call on you to facilitate communication between patient and provider. This patient, at the time you arrive at the appointment, is sitting outside the consultation room. As he sees you, he asks if you are the interpreter, and he starts sharing with you how he is feeling and that he has been having suicidal thoughts. You, as the appointed interpreter to this consultation, are concerned about the patient's well-being. Discuss the ethical issues involved from the two perspectives: yours (the perspective of a freelance interpreter sent by an agency/the government language service/staff member of the HO) and the medical intern's (psychiatric perspective). What would you do about the information you are receiving in the waiting room? Do you leave with an excuse (e.g. you need to make a phone call)? Do you stop the patient and explain what you have to do with the information you are receiving? Are you afraid of the patient's reaction? Are you concerned about violating his trust? What do you see as conflicting or converging views between you and the medical intern? What do you think you should do next? Go into the consultation and interpret? Reveal the information you received to the medical intern? If so, would you do it before or after the medical consultation? Would you forget about the information you received in the waiting room?

Let us assume that you see it as your duty to inform the medical intern about what you heard in confidence. You do this because you are mostly concerned about the health of the patient. If you have a chance, you may ask questions of the patient to understand his concern, but you realize it is not up to you to give advice. At the same time, you also realize that by informing the medical intern, you may violate the patient's confidentiality. You are assessing the impact on the trust that the patient is putting on you. You know that once the information is revealed, the patient may be upset and complain about your work. You may even be at risk of losing your job as a result of the complaint. You need to determine whether there is some degree of flexibility in deciding what information, if any, you can share with the healthcare provider. Your code of ethics is clear about your responsibilities, and you cannot breach the clause of confidentiality. How are you going to proceed? Write down your plan of action, state the reasons for it and find support for your decision in codes of ethics.

Scenario 2: You are called to interpret between a general practitioner who speaks the societal language (YY) and a patient who shares your language (XX) during a consultation. The patient is suffering from nausea and shortness of breath. The doctor has seen this patient several times. During this encounter the doctor reminds the patient that he will not get any better if he does not take the medication. In so doing, you notice the doctor is quite harsh on the patient.

As the interpreter, you suspect that the patient does not take the medication as indicated because of a cultural difference. You know that, because of tradition, the patient does not trust the Western HCP and prefers to treat himself with the herbs recommended by the home "doctor." You know that the doctor is already upset with this patient because it seems that nothing of what he said in the past has been implemented. You are the only person who understands the situation. You have various options: you simply interpret the exchanges between the HCP and the patient, knowing well that the patient will do whatever he feels best for him. Or you explain to the doctor what the issue is, so that he starts explaining things in a way that the patient might understand. As an interpreter, you feel that you have contributed to a better understanding, beyond the words. The doctor will realize that there may be more than one way to do things, especially in intercultural healthcare. Maybe he will be able to put this into good use for the future. He too, as yourself as interpreter, will evaluate the outcome and consider what might be done differently next time.

Scenario 3: You are interpreting between a female in her forties and an OBGYN male doctor assisted by an OBGYN nurse. The patient speaks your language. The patient came with her three children: the eldest boy is five, and the two twins (a boy and a girl) are three. The patient is pregnant in her sixth month. As the family came into the room and the patient greeted the doctor and the nurse, the patient addressed the interpreter directly to apologize for bringing the children to the visit. The patient explained she planned to have a sitter at home to take care of the children, but the friend who was supposed to come to the house canceled at the last minute. The patient also explained that because it has been difficult to get an appointment, she preferred to bring the children with her rather than to cancel. You interpret all of this information to the doctor and the consultation starts.

You notice the children sitting on the examination table, giggling and being loud. They start taking out books and colored pencils. The mother tries to keep them quiet and at times it is difficult to hear. You change positions in the room and get further away from the children. You continue working in spite of the noise and ask for repetition/clarification when necessary. At one point, the doctor asks the patient to lie on the table so that he could examine her better.

This means the children are asked to get off the bed. As they start gathering their books and jackets, they push each other to get to the chairs first and the mother scolds them. During the examination, the doctor makes the following comment to the nurse in YY: "I do not understand why these people would like to have more children if they cannot control the ones they already have." The nurse does not respond and the consultation goes on.

Once the consultation concludes, the mother says goodbye and apologizes for the children's behavior. Your interpreting assignment concludes then. You say goodbye to the doctor and nurse and leave immediately after the patient.

What are your thoughts about what you witnessed? The comment was not interpreted. If you needed to justify this decision on your part, what would you say? What do you think you should do with the information you have?

As the interpreter for the encounter, while all of the above was happening, you were considering various alternatives. You could remain silent during the interaction, as you did. It has the advantage of avoiding a potential cultural clash and an uncomfortable situation for the patient and for the doctor. Things could escalate if the patient were to exercise her right of complaint for discrimination. You determine that by withholding that information you are not putting the patient at risk and you are not withholding crucial information for the doctor to be able to provide quality care for the patient. By not contributing to what potentially would become a difficult situation, you retain the doctor's trust as you did not expose him, but you feel you have hidden some information to which the patient was entitled. The benefit of not saying anything to the patient is that you have ensured that the consultation continued without stress or anger.

Another possibility is that you interpret for the patient exactly what you heard. After all, this is exactly what you heard and you are there to interpret. Because this was a comment made in English directly to the physician's colleague who was with him assisting in the room (the nurse), you are aware that interpreting the derogatory remark by the provider does not contribute much to the communication between the patient and the provider, and that you may actually be adding to the tension.

Options of taking action after the fact include the following:

1 You might also decide to speak to the provider at the end of the consultation and tell him that such remarks can be offensive, that you have decided not to interpret it but that behaviors like this one put you in an awkward position vis-à-vis the patient and put you at risk of not being asked to interpret anymore for this doctor. The advantage is that the patient will continue to trust you and the provider, alerted by you, may choose in the future a culturally more appropriate way to discuss. This would be a win-win situation. Alternatively, you may decide to report the provider to the office of patient's services/advocacy or to report directly to the social workers' office.
2 You might talk to the patient and explain how you feel; that it is your duty to interpret everything you hear and is pertinent to the case; that they should refrain from telling things that should not be interpreted.

References

Abraham, D., Cabral N., & Tancredi, A. (Eds.). *A handbook for trainers: Language interpreting in the healthcare sector.* Toronto: Healthcare Interpretation Network.

Angelelli, C. V. (2015). *A study on public service translation in cross-border healthcare: Technical report.* Luxembourg: Publications Office of the European Union. ISBN 978-92-79-47163-6.

———. (2007a). Accommodating the need for medical interpreters: The California endowment interpreter testing project (This work was made possible by The California Endowment Grant G00005318). *The Translator*, *13*(1), 63–82.

———. (2007b). Validating professional standards and codes: Challenges and opportunities. *Interpreting: International Journal of Research and Practice in Interpreting*, *8*(2), 175–193.

Bankauskaite, V., & Jakusovaite, I. (2006). Dealing with ethical problems in the healthcare system in Lithuania: Achievements and challenges. *Journal of Medical Ethics*, *32*(10), 584–587. http://doi.org/10.1136/jme.2005.014761

Bauer, H. M., Rodriguez, M. A., Szkupinski Quiroga, S., & Flores-Ortiz, Y. G. (2000). Barriers to health care for abused Latina and Asian immigrant women. *Journal of Health Care for the Poor & Underserved*, *11*(1), 33–44.

Cambridge, J. (1999). Information loss in bilingual medical interviews through an untrained interpreter. *The Translator*, *5*, 201–219.

Chan, A., & Woodruff, R. K. (1999). Comparison of palliative care needs of English- and non-English-speaking patients. *Journal of Palliative Care*, *15*(1), 26–30.

CHIA (California Healthcare Interpreters Association). (2002). *California standards for healthcare interpreters: Ethical principles, protocols, and guidance on roles and intervention.* Sacramento: California Endowment.

Davidson, B. (2000). The interpreter as institutional gatekeeper: The social-linguistic role of interpreters in Spanish-English medical discourse. *Journal of Sociolinguistics*, *4*(3), 379–405.

Flores, G., Barton Laws, M., & Mayo, S. J., Zuckerman, B., Abreu, M., Medina, L., & Hardt, E. J. (2003). Errors in medical interpretation and their potential clinical consequences in pediatric encounters. *Pediatrics*, *111*(1), 6–14.

Health21. (1999). The health for all policy framework for the WHO European region. *The Journal of Advanced Nursing*, *30*(2), 280. Available at Pubmed www.ncbi.nlm.nih.gov/pubmed/10484702 (Last accessed April, 2018).

Hlavac, J. (2010). Ethical implications in situations where the language of interpretation shifts: The AUSIT code of ethics re-visited. *Translation & Interpreting*, *2*(2), 29–43.

Hsieh, E., & Kramer, E. M. (2012). Medical interpreters as tools: Dangers and challenges in the utilitarian approach to interpreters' roles and functions. *Patient Education and Counseling*, *89*(1), 158–162. http://doi.org/10.1016/j.pec.2012.07.001

IMIA. (2006). International Medical Interpreting Association Code of Ethics. Available at www.imiaweb.org/code/ (Last accessed May, 2018).

Ko, L. (2006). "Fine-tuning the code of ethics for interpreters and translators" In S. M. Rogers (Ed.), *Informed performance: Professional Development, Communion & Ethics*, *2*(3).

National Council for Interpreters in Healthcare. (2004). Available at www.ncihc.org/assets/documents/publications/NCIHC%20National%20Code%20of%20Ethics.pdf (Last accessed May, 2018).

National Registry of Public Service Interpreters Code of Professional Conduct. (2016). Available at www.nrpsi.org.uk/downloads/NRPSI_Code_of_Professional_Conduct_22.01.16.pdf (Last accessed May, 2018).

Official Journal of the European Union. (2011). Directive 2011/24/EU of the European Parliament and of the Council of 9 March 2011 on the application of patients' rights in cross-border healthcare. *European Union* (Ed.), *54*. Luxembourg: Publications Office of the European Union.

———. (2004). *Regulation (EC) No 883/2004 of the European Parliament and of the Council of 29 April 2004*. Luxembourg: Publications Office of the European Union.

Rassin, M. (2008). Nurses' professional and personal values. *Nursing Ethics*, *15*(5), 614–630. https://doi.org/10.1177/0969733008092870

Riddick, F. (2003). The code of medical ethics of the American Medical Association. *The Ochsner Journal*, *5*, 6–10.

Swabey, L., & Mickelson, P. (2008). Role definition: A perspective on forty years of professionalism in sign language interpreting. In C. Valero-Garces & A. Martin (Eds.), *Crossing borders in community interpreting* (pp. 51–80). Amsterdam and Philadelphia: John Benjamins Publishing Company.

Further readings and resources

Further readings

Bosch, Y. V. (2005). Accuracy of the interpretation and translation: Integrity and ethics, monitoring of recordings of proceedings, and professional code of ethics. In W. J. Gasille & H. Keijzer-Lambooy (Eds.), *Aequilibrium: Instruments for lifting language barriers in intercultural legal proceedings*. EU Project Report JAI/2003/AUIS/048, Ultrecht: ITV Hogeschool voor Tolken en vertalen (Last accessed 15 March 2019 at: https://core.ac.uk/download/pdf/34556039.pdf).

Corsellis, A., & Fernández, L. F. (2001). Code of ethics and conduct and guidelines to good practice. In E. Hertog (Ed.), *Aequitas: Access to justice across language and culture in the EU*. EU project Report. Chapter 7 (Last accessed 15 March 2019 at: https://eulita.eu/wp/wp-content/uploads/files/Aequitas_Acces%20to%20Justice%20across%20Language%20and%20Culture%20in%20the%20EU.pdf)

NHS England. Principles for high quality interpreting and translation services. Available at www.england.nhs.uk/commissioning/wp-content/uploads/sites/12/2015/03/it_principles.pdf (Last accessed May 15, 2018).

Valero, C. (2005). Emotional and psychological effects on interpreters in public services. A critical factor to bear in mind. Available at en www.accurapid.com/jounal/33ips.htm

Verrept, H. (2008). Intercultural mediation: An answer to health care disparities? In C. Valero Garcés & A. Martin (Eds.), *Crossing borders in community interpreting: Definitions and dilemmas*. Amsterdam and Philadelphia: Benjamins.

Further resources

Examples of code of ethics and standards of practice for healthcare interpreters

1 Australia

AUSIT. Australia Code of Ethics for Interpreters and Translators (2012). https://ausit.org/AUSIT/Documents/Code_Of_Ethics_Full.pdf

2 The Netherlands

Dutch Association for Sign Language Interpreters (NBTG): Code of Ethics for Sign Language Interpreters Available at: www.nbtg.nl/sites/default/files/1403%20Code%20of%20Ethics.pdf (last accessed November 2014).

3 United Kingdom

- National Registry of Public Service Interpreters Code of Professional Conduct (2016)
- Northern Ireland Health and Social Services Interpreting Service, *Code of Ethics and Good Practice Guidelines for Interpreters*: www.saludycultura.uji.es/archivos/NIHSSIS_CoE_and_Good_Practice_for_Interpreters_(NIreland).pdf

4 United States

- California Healthcare Interpreting Association. (2002). *California standards for healthcare interpreters: Ethical principles, protocols, and guidance on roles and intervention*. Sacramento: California Endowment. www.chiaonline.org/CHIA-Standards (last accessed May 2018).
- IMIA 2006. International Medical Interpreting Association Code of Ethics. First established in 1987 and revised in 2006. www.imiaweb.org/code/ (last accessed May 2018).
- National Council for Interpreters in Healthcare 2004 www.ncihc.org/assets/documents/publications/NCIHC%20National%20Code%20of%20Ethics.pdf

Examples of codes for linguistic/cultural mediators (Italy)

Cooperativa Sociale Kantara, *Codice di comportamento del mediatore linguistico culturale*: www.kantara.it/home.asp?sezione=7

(www.saludycultura.uji.es/archivos/CODIGO_COMPORTAMIENTO_MEDIACION_(KANTARA).pdf) (last accessed June 2018).

Useful websites/reference materials

Multi-Languages Corporation *Code of Ethics Interpreters*, accessed on 1 May 2018 at https://multi-languages.com/interpretations-shtml/interpreters_ethics-shtml/. The *National Standard Guide for Community Interpreting Services* is an initiative of the Healthcare Interpretation Network – HIN in collaboration with AILIA, ACCTI and CLC (Canada).

NAJIT (2003). *Code of Ethics and Professional Responsibilities*. www.najit.org/ethics.html

National Council for Interpreters in Healthcare. www.ncihc.org/resources

Pharos. Centre of expertise on health disparities in the Netherlands: www.pharos.nl/information-in-english/about-us

SALUDyCULTURA (website about cross-cultural communication in a healthcare setting. Research group Grupo CRIT, Universitat Jaume I de Castelló, Spain): www.saludycultura.uji.es/index.php

Looking ahead

As we come to the end of our journey, we look back at what we have accomplished and we look ahead to see what comes next. Together we have explored the basic concepts of healthcare interpreting, a complex situated practice that has been evolving rapidly in the last 20 years.

We started our journey learning and reflecting about the professional practice of healthcare interpreting. We have discussed the settings where healthcare interpreters work, the parties with whom they interact and the different ways in which they express themselves to discuss issues. We paid special attention to both content and form of interactions. We reflected on learning and acquiring both the receptive and productive skills necessary to perform interpreting and accomplish communication across languages. In addition, we explored some of the social factors that impact communication as both main interlocutors engage in achieving their communicative goals. We looked at the various roles interpreters play, the dilemmas they face and the ethical principles to which they turn for guidance.

Each of the chapters offered us opportunities to reflect, research and explore more on the topics and on our thoughts on (as well as our reactions to) the materials discussed. Once we gained an understanding of the profession, the research, the learning and teaching of healthcare interpreting and the practice, the time has come to direct our attention to what comes next.

We have discussed the value of exploring professional associations and meeting colleagues. The time has come now for you to decide what steps you will be taking to put this knowledge to work. Whether you decide to explore further educational or training opportunities in healthcare interpreting or a related field (e.g. human resource manager, project manager), take a certification exam to obtain a credential you can show to validate your work as interpreter, or turn to your professional association for guidance on opportunities in your area; you have several options from which to choose. Healthcare interpreters may work either as staff members or freelancers. They may work face-to-face or remotely (via telephone or videoconferencing). Some of the interpreters are also interested in managing projects (e.g. multilingual medical databases) or managing a unit of interpreting/language services in a hospital, for example.

In many of our societies, language and cultural diversity is more the norm than the exception. For human beings, few things matter more in life than maintaining good health or recovering it. As this book explains, languages are not barriers. Users of different languages do not pose a risk to healthcare. What we, as a society, do with different languages is what matters. Healthcare interpreting affords all of us equal opportunities to access healthcare. Healthcare interpreting bridges language and cultural diversity. Therefore, opportunities are countless for healthcare interpreters who will successfully bridge differences to enable all members of society access to healthcare across languages. We hope that this book and our work together have inspired you to pursue a career in a field which is both demanding and rewarding.

Glossary

Applied linguistics an interdisciplinary field of inquiry focusing on language-related real-life problems (e.g. language in communication, language learning/testing, translation and interpreting).

Balanced bilingual a person with almost equal competency in L1 and L2.

Cross-border healthcare EU citizens can pursue healthcare across borders; they can access healthcare in any of the member states of the European Union.

Cultural mediators a person that mediates between two cultural groups defined by language, origin, profession, among other social factors (e.g. Spanish and French; doctors and patients).

Dialogue interpreting interpreting between two persons, generally in short consecutive.

Healthcare interpreting used interchangeably most of the time with medical interpreting.

Interpreting agencies company that manages freelance or employed interpreters and sends them off to assignments with companies/organizations with which the agency has agreements/contracts.

Language register level of formality of a language; different contexts, situations or people may require the use of different registers (e.g. interacting with a child, working with a court officer in a mental health ward).

Liaison interpreting interpreting between two parties who speak/sign different languages, usually without the use of equipment, often performed in short consecutive.

Linguistic minorities groups that cannot access the societal language of the region where they live.

Medical interpreting interpreting in a medical context. See *healthcare interpreting*.

Medical tourism traveling to another country/region with the main goal of accessing healthcare for treatment, surgery and so forth.

Morbidity the condition of being diseased, ill or unhealthy.

Palliative care special type of care for people with serious illnesses; it focuses on relieving stress, pain and symptoms.

Patient compliance refers to the degree to which a patient follows medical advice.

Public-service interpreting term used in Europe to refer to interpreting that occurs when speakers of non-societal languages (linguistic minorities) need to access services such as healthcare, education or justice. This is also called community interpreting.

Short consecutive interpreting rendered after the source is spoken or signed. Because the chunks of spoken or signed language are small, notes are generally not taken. The interpreter asks for pauses or uses natural pauses to render the interpreted meaning.

Sight translation the interpreter renders the written document in one language into another oral or signed language. The input is a written text and the output is a spoken/signed rendition of such text.

Situated practice interpreting, like other practices, is shaped by a specific context and a variety of social and other factors present in such context.

Societal language the language used by the majority of speakers in a specific society/region.

Sociolinguistics A field of inquiry, a science focusing on language and society (e.g. language policy, language planning, language discrimination). It studies language in relation to society. The object of study is language.

Speech act an utterance that has a specific function in communication (e.g. an apology, a request, a complaint, an insult, a joke).

Speech community a community that shares the same ways of speaking/signing, speech characteristics and ways of interpreting meanings (e.g. aristocrats, rappers, lawyers, football players). Community members are all familiar with these ways and forms of speaking/signing.

Speech event a speech during a situation (e.g. a speech during a party).

Speech situation a ceremony, fight, meal, party.

Index